ANTI-INFLAMMATORY RECIPES

"Healthy and Anti-inflammatory Cooking with 100 Delicious Recipes to Reduce Inflammation"

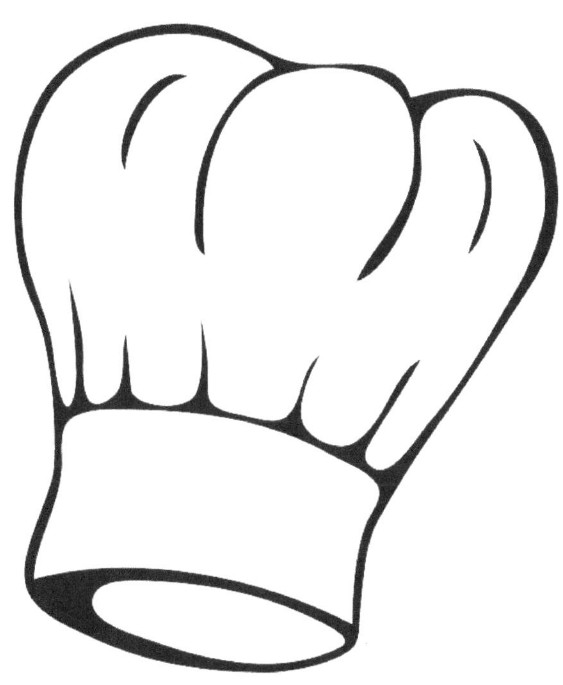

INDEX

Introduction

Inflammation is a natural response of our body to some aggressions or imbalances. However, when it becomes chronic it can be the source of numerous health problems, from allergies and arthritis to obesity and some types of cancer.

Luckily, it is proven that an adequate diet plays a key role in the prevention and control of this type of inflammation. In this book I present 100 recipes with anti-inflammatory ingredients and properties to help you improve your quality of life.

Thanks to the advice of expert nutritionists and chefs, I have selected easy-to-follow preparations that will help reduce pain, swelling, fatigue and other common symptoms of inflammatory processes. All our recipes are nutritious, tasty, and suitable for different tastes and special diets.

With this complete recipe book, you will discover a new world of gastronomic possibilities to implement a healthy, varied, and anti-inflammatory diet. I invite you to join this journey towards well-being, vitality, and good eating. Enjoy these delicious foods that, in addition to nourishing, help us heal.

Kale and avocado salad

Ingredients:

- 1 large bunch of kale

- 2 ripe avocados

- 1/2 cup of walnuts (you can use walnuts, almonds, or pine nuts)

- 1/2 cup raisins or dried cranberries

- 2 tablespoons of fresh lemon juice

- 2 tablespoons of olive oil

- Salt and freshly ground black pepper

Instructions:

1) Wash the kale well and dry it with a paper towel. Remove the thick stems and cut the leaves into small pieces.

2) Put the kale in a large bowl and add 1 tablespoon olive oil, 1 tablespoon lemon juice, salt, and black pepper to taste. Mix everything well and massage the kale with your hands to soften it a little.

3) Cut the avocados in half, remove the stone, and peel the pulp. Cut the avocado flesh into cubes and add it to the bowl with the kale.

4) Add the walnuts and raisins or dried cranberries to the salad and mix everything gently.

5) In a small bowl, mix 1 tablespoon of olive oil and 1 tablespoon of lemon juice. Add salt and black pepper to taste and mix well.

6) Pour the olive oil and lemon mixture over the salad and mix everything well.

7) Serve the salad and enjoy.

Preparation time: 15 to 20 minutes.

Servings: 4

Beet and orange salad

Ingredients:

• 4 medium beets, cooked and peeled

• 2 medium oranges, peeled and cut into thin slices

• 1/2 cup fresh mint leaves, chopped

• 1/4 cup chopped walnuts (you can use walnuts, almonds, or pistachios)

• 2 tablespoons of red wine vinegar

• 2 tablespoons of olive oil

• Salt and freshly ground black pepper

Instructions:

1) Cut the beets into cubes or thin slices and place them in a large bowl.

2) Add the orange slices and chopped mint leaves to the bowl with the beets.

3) Add the chopped walnuts to the salad and mix everything gently.

4) In a small container, mix the red wine vinegar and olive oil. Add salt and black pepper to taste and mix well.

5) Pour the vinegar and oil mixture over the salad and mix everything well.

6) Serve the salad and enjoy.

Preparation time: Approximately 20 to 25 minutes, depending on how long it takes you to cook and peel the beets.

Servings: 4

Grilled fish with tomato and basil sauce

Ingredients:

- 4 fish fillets (you can use salmon, trout, tilapia, or any white fish)

- 2 cups of chopped tomatoes

- 1/4 cup fresh basil leaves, chopped

- 2 cloves of garlic, minced

- 2 tablespoons of olive oil

- Salt and freshly ground black pepper

1 lemon, cut into quarters

Instructions:

1) Preheat the grill to medium-high heat.

2) In a small bowl, mix together the chopped tomatoes, chopped basil leaves, minced garlic and olive oil. Add salt and black pepper to taste and mix well.

3) Place the fish fillets on the grill and cook for 3-4 minutes on each side, depending on the thickness of the fish.

4) Once the fish fillets are cooked, remove them from the grill and place them on a plate.

5) Pour the tomato and basil sauce over the fish fillets and serve with the lemon quarters on the side.

Preparation time: Approximately 20 to 25 minutes

Fish tacos with pineapple and cilantro sauce

Ingredients:

- 1 pound fish fillets (you can use tilapia, mahi mahi or any other white fish)

- 1 tablespoon olive oil

- 1 tablespoon fresh lemon juice

- 1 teaspoon chili powder

- 1/2 teaspoon ground cumin

- 1/2 teaspoon salt

- 8 corn tortillas

- 1 cup chopped fresh pineapple

- 1/4 cup chopped fresh cilantro

- 1/4 cup chopped red onion

- 1/4 cup nonfat Greek yogurt

Instructions:

1) Preheat oven to 375 degrees F (190 degrees C).

2) Place the fish fillets on a baking sheet. Drizzle the fillets with olive oil and lemon juice.

3) In a small bowl, mix together the chili powder, cumin and salt. Sprinkle the spice mixture over the fish fillets.

4) Bake the fish fillets for 15-20 minutes or until cooked.

5) While the fish is cooking, heat the tortillas in a hot skillet for about 30 seconds on each side.

6) In a small bowl, mix together the chopped pineapple, chopped cilantro, chopped red onion, and nonfat Greek yogurt. Add salt to taste.

7) When the fish fillets are cooked, cut the fillets into bite-sized pieces.

8) Place the fish pieces on each tortilla and cover with the pineapple and cilantro sauce.

Preparation time: Approximately 30 to 35 minutes

Servings: 4

Grilled chicken with broccoli and almond salad

Ingredients:

- 4 boneless, skinless chicken breasts

- 1 tablespoon olive oil

- Salt and ground black pepper to taste

- 4 cups fresh broccoli florets

- 1/2 cup slivered almonds

- 1/4 cup chopped red onion

- 1/4 cup apple cider vinegar

- 2 tablespoons Dijon mustard

- 2 tablespoons of honey

- 1 tablespoon olive oil

- Juice of half a lemon

Instructions:

1) Preheat the grill to medium-high heat.

2) Brush the chicken breasts with olive oil and season with salt and black pepper to taste. Place the chicken breasts on the grill and cook for about 6-8 minutes on each side or until golden brown and cooked through.

3) Meanwhile, in a small frying pan, toast the slivered almonds over medium heat for 2-3 minutes, stirring constantly until golden.

4) In a large bowl, mix the broccoli florets, chopped red onion, and toasted almonds.

5) In a small bowl, whisk together the apple cider vinegar, Dijon mustard, honey, olive oil, and lemon juice. Beat until well combined.

6) Pour the dressing mixture over the broccoli salad and mix well.

7) Serve the grilled chicken breasts with the broccoli and almond salad.

Preparation time: Approximately 30 to 35 minutes

Servings: 4!

Lentil curry with pumpkin and spinach

Ingredients:

- 1 cup of dried lentils

- 4 cups of water

- 1 tablespoon olive oil

- 1 medium onion chopped

- 3 cloves of garlic, minced

- 1 tablespoon grated fresh ginger

- 1 tablespoon red curry paste

- 1 tablespoon of ground cumin

- 1 tablespoon of ground coriander

- 1 tablespoon turmeric powder

- 1 can of 400 grams of peeled tomatoes

- 1 cup of vegetable broth

- 2 cups of pumpkin cut into cubes

- 2 cups fresh spinach leaves

- Salt and ground black pepper to taste

- Fresh lemon juice to serve

- Chopped fresh cilantro to decorate

Instructions:

1) Rinse the dried lentils in cold water and drain. Put them in a saucepan with 4 cups of water and bring to a boil over medium heat. Reduce heat and simmer until lentils are tender, about 20-25 minutes. Drain the water and reserve the cooked lentils.

2) Heat the olive oil in a large pot over medium-high heat. Add the chopped onion and cook until golden brown, about 3-4 minutes. Add the minced garlic and grated ginger and cook for another 2 minutes.

3) Add the red curry paste, ground cumin, ground coriander and turmeric powder to the pot and cook for a further 2-3 minutes, stirring constantly.

4) Add the peeled tomatoes and vegetable broth to the pot and mix well. Bring to a boil and reduce heat to medium-low. Cover the pot and cook for 10 minutes, stirring occasionally.

5) Add the diced squash to the pot and cook for another 10-15 minutes or until the squash is tender.

6) Add the cooked lentils and fresh spinach leaves to the pot and cook for another 2-3 minutes, stirring gently until the spinach has wilted.

7) Season with salt and black pepper to taste.

8) Serve the pumpkin and spinach lentil curry with a little lemon juice and fresh chopped cilantro on top.

Preparation time: 45 minutes

Servings: 4

Brown rice with vegetable curry

Ingredients:

- 2 cups of brown rice

- 4 cups of water

- 1 chopped onion

- 2 cloves of garlic, minced

- 1 tablespoon grated fresh ginger

- 2 carrots peeled and cut into small cubes

- 1 zucchini cut into small cubes

- 1 red pepper cut into small cubes

- 1 tablespoon curry powder

- 1/2 teaspoon cumin powder

- 1/2 teaspoon turmeric powder

- 1/4 teaspoon cinnamon powder

- Salt and pepper to taste

- Olive oil

To decorate:

- Chopped fresh cilantro

- Sliced almonds

Instructions:

1) Rinse the brown rice and place it in a pot with the water. Bring to a boil, reduce heat, and cook, covered, for 45-50 minutes, until the water has been completely absorbed and the rice is tender. Remove from heat and let sit for 10 minutes.

2) Meanwhile, heat a large skillet over medium-high heat. Add a little olive oil and sauté the onion, garlic, and ginger for 2-3 minutes until golden and fragrant.

3) Add the carrots, zucchini and red pepper to the pan and sauté for about 5 minutes, until tender.

4) Add the curry powder, cumin, turmeric, cinnamon, salt, and pepper to the pan and mix well with the vegetables.

5) Add 1/2 cup water to the pan and simmer for 10-15 minutes, until the vegetables are tender, and the sauce has thickened slightly.

6) Serve the brown rice on individual plates and add the vegetable mixture on top. Garnish with fresh chopped cilantro and slivered almonds.

Preparation time: 15 minutes.

Cooking time: 1 hour.

Servings: 4 people.

Lentil and vegetable soup

Ingredients:

• 1 cup of dried lentils

• 1 chopped onion

• 2 cloves of garlic, minced

• 2 carrots peeled and cut into cubes

• 2 stalks of celery, chopped

• 1 red pepper cut into cubes

• 4 cups of vegetable broth

• 1 teaspoon ground cumin

• 1 teaspoon paprika

• Salt and pepper to taste

• Olive oil

• Lemon juice

• Chopped fresh cilantro

Instructions:

1) Rinse the lentils and soak them in water for at least 1 hour.

2) In a large pot, heat some olive oil over medium heat. Add the onion and garlic and cook for a few minutes until soft.

3) Add the carrots, celery, and red pepper, and cook for a few more minutes until soft.

4) Add the drained lentils, vegetable broth, cumin and paprika. Mix everything well and bring to a boil.

5) Reduce heat and simmer until lentils are soft, approximately 30 to 40 minutes.

6) Add salt and pepper to taste.

7) Serve hot and add a splash of lime juice and fresh chopped cilantro before serving.

Preparation time: Approximately 1 hour and 15 minutes (including soaking the lentils)

Servings: 4

Tomato and basil soup

Ingredients:

- 2 tablespoons of olive oil

- 1 chopped onion

- 3 cloves of garlic, minced

- 4 cups of fresh tomatoes, peeled and chopped

- 4 cups of chicken or vegetable broth

- 1/2 cup fresh basil leaves

- 1 tablespoon of brown sugar

- Salt and pepper to taste

Instructions:

1) Heat the olive oil in a large pot over medium-high heat. Add the onion and garlic and sauté until golden and fragrant, about 5 minutes.

2) Add the chopped tomatoes to the pot and sauté for another 5 minutes.

3) Add the chicken or vegetable broth to the pot and bring the soup to a boil. Reduce the heat and let the soup simmer for about 20-25 minutes.

4) Add the basil leaves and brown sugar to the soup. Stir well and cook for another 5 minutes.

5) Remove the soup from the heat and let it cool slightly. Then, blend the soup in a blender or food processor until smooth and creamy.

6) Reheat the soup over medium heat and season with salt and pepper to taste.

Serve hot with fresh basil leaves and bread croutons if desired.

Preparation time: 45 minutes

Servings: 4 people

Beet and quinoa salad

Ingredients:

• 2 cups of cooked quinoa

• 2 medium beets cooked and chopped

• 1/2 cup chopped walnuts

• 1/4 cup olive oil

• 2 tablespoons balsamic vinegar

• 1 teaspoon of honey

• Salt and pepper to taste

• Lettuce leaves to decorate

Instructions:

1) In a large bowl, mix the cooked quinoa, beets and chopped walnuts.

2) In another small bowl, whisk together the olive oil, balsamic vinegar, honey, salt, and pepper until well combined.

3) Pour the dressing over the quinoa and beet mixture and mix well.

4) Serve on salad plates decorated with lettuce leaves.

Preparation time: Approximately 20-25 minutes if the quinoa and beets are already cooked.

Servings: 4 people

Walnut crusted baked salmon

Ingredients:

- 4 salmon fillets

- 1 cup chopped walnuts

- 1/4 cup breadcrumbs

- 2 tablespoons of olive oil

- 2 tablespoons Dijon mustard

- 2 tablespoons of honey

- 2 tablespoons of lemon juice

- Salt and pepper to taste

At your service:

- Lemon slices

Instructions:

1) Preheat the oven to 200°C.

2) Mix the chopped walnuts and breadcrumbs in a bowl.

3) In another bowl, mix the olive oil, Dijon mustard, honey and lemon juice.

4) Season the salmon fillets with salt and pepper to taste.

5) Place the salmon fillets on a baking sheet.

6) Spread the mustard mixture over the salmon fillets.

7) Cover the salmon fillets with the walnut and breadcrumb mixture.

8) Bake for 12-15 minutes, or until the salmon is cooked and the walnut crust is golden brown.

9) Serve with lemon slices.

Preparation time: 15 minutes

Cooking time: 15 minutes

Servings: 4 people

<u>Baked chicken with turmeric and lemon</u>

Ingredients:

• 4 boneless, skinless chicken breasts

• 2 tablespoons of olive oil

• 1 teaspoon turmeric

• 1/2 teaspoon ground cumin

• 1/2 teaspoon smoked paprika

• 1/4 teaspoon ground cinnamon

• Salt and ground black pepper, to taste

• 2 lemons, one for juice and one to cut into thin slices

• 4 cloves of garlic, peeled and crushed

• 1 large red onion, cut into thin slices

Instructions:

1) Preheat the oven to 200°C.

2) In a small bowl, mix the olive oil, turmeric, cumin, smoked paprika, cinnamon, salt, and pepper to taste. Add the juice of one lemon and mix well.

3) Place the chicken breasts on a baking sheet and brush with the spice mixture.

4) Arrange the lemon slices, crushed garlic cloves, and onion slices over the chicken.

5) Bake the chicken for 25-30 minutes, or until completely cooked.

6) Serve the chicken with the grilled lemon and onion slices on top.

Preparation time: 10 minutes

Cooking time: 25-30 minutes

Servings: 4 people.

Smoked salmon salad with avocado and cucumber

Ingredients:

• 4 cups chopped romaine lettuce

• 1 large cucumber, peeled and cut into cubes

• 1 ripe avocado, peeled and cut into cubes

• 1/2 red onion chopped

• 4 ounces smoked salmon, shredded

• 2 tablespoons of fresh lemon juice

• 2 tablespoons of olive oil

• Salt and pepper to taste

Instructions:

1) In a large bowl, combine lettuce, cucumber, avocado and red onion. Mix well.

2) Add the crumbled smoked salmon and mix gently.

3) In a small bowl, mix the lemon juice, olive oil, salt, and pepper.

4) Pour the lemon mixture over the salad and mix well.

5) Serve the smoked salmon salad with avocado and cucumber and enjoy.

Preparation time: 15 minutes.

Servings: 4 people

Stir-fried tofu with vegetables and ginger

Ingredients:

• 400g firm tofu

• 2 tablespoons of olive oil

• 1 chopped onion

• 3 cloves of garlic, minced

• 1 tablespoon grated fresh ginger

• 1 red pepper in strips

• 1 green pepper in strips

• 1 cup sliced mushrooms

• 1 carrot in thin strips

• 2 tablespoons soy sauce

• 1 teaspoon brown sugar

• Salt and pepper to taste

• Chopped chives to decorate

Instructions:

1) Cut the tofu into medium-sized cubes and pat dry with a paper towel. Booking.

2) In a large skillet or wok, heat the olive oil over medium-high heat.

3) Add the onion, garlic and ginger, and sauté until golden.

4) Add the peppers, mushrooms, and carrot, and continue sautéing for a few minutes until the vegetables are cooked but still crisp.

5) Add the tofu to the pan and mix well with the vegetables.

6) In a small bowl, mix soy sauce, brown sugar, salt, and pepper.

7) Pour the soy sauce mixture over the tofu and vegetables and stir until everything is well coated.

8) Continue cooking over medium-high heat for a few more minutes, until the tofu is golden brown, and the vegetables are tender, but still crisp.

9) Serve hot and decorate with chopped chives.

Preparation time: 20 minutes.

Servings: 4 people.

Salmon burgers with cucumber and mint salad

Ingredients:

• 500 grams of salmon fillet without skin or bones

• 1/4 cup breadcrumbs

• 1 beaten egg

• 1/4 cup chopped onion

• 2 tablespoons Dijon mustard

- 2 tablespoons chopped fresh parsley

- 1 tablespoon lemon zest

- 1/2 teaspoon salt

- 1/4 teaspoon ground black pepper

- 4 hamburger buns

- 1/2 cup Greek yogurt

- 1/4 cup chopped cucumber

- 1/4 cup chopped mint leaves

- 1/2 teaspoon salt

- 1/4 teaspoon ground black pepper

Instructions:

1) Preheat the oven to 200°C.

2) Cut the salmon into small pieces and place in a food processor. Blend until chopped into small pieces, but not completely ground.

3) In a large bowl, combine the chopped salmon with the breadcrumbs, beaten egg, chopped onion, Dijon mustard, chopped fresh parsley, lemon zest, salt, and ground black pepper. Mix well.

4) Form four burgers with the salmon mixture.

5) Heat a large skillet over medium-high heat. Add the salmon burgers and cook for 2-3 minutes on each side or until golden brown.

6) Transfer the salmon burgers to a baking sheet and place in the preheated oven. Cook for 8-10 minutes or until completely cooked.

7) Meanwhile, in a small bowl, mix Greek yogurt, chopped cucumber, chopped mint leaves, salt and ground black pepper to make the salad.

8) Once the salmon burgers are ready, remove from the oven and let rest for 5 minutes.

9) Place the salmon burgers on the hamburger buns and serve with the cucumber and mint salad.

Preparation time: 20 minutes

Cooking time: 15 minutes

Servings: 4 people.

Lentil and brown rice salad

Ingredients:

- 1 cup of cooked brown rice

- 1 cup of cooked lentils

- 1 red pepper cut into small cubes

- 1 red onion cut into small cubes

- 2 medium carrots cut into small cubes

- 1/2 cup sweet corn

- 1/4 cup olive oil

- 2 tablespoons of red wine vinegar

- 1 teaspoon Dijon mustard

- 1 clove of garlic, minced

- Salt and pepper to taste

- Lettuce or spinach leaves to serve

Instructions:

1) Cook the brown rice and lentils separately, following package instructions. Once cooked, place them in a large bowl and mix well.

2) Add the red pepper, red onion, carrots and corn to the rice and lentil mixture. Stir everything to combine.

3) In a small bowl, whisk together the olive oil, red wine vinegar, Dijon mustard, and minced garlic. Beat well until the mixture is smooth and uniform.

4) Pour the dressing mixture over the rice and lentil salad and mix well to coat all the ingredients.

5) Add salt and pepper to taste and mix again.

6) Serve the lentil and brown rice salad on lettuce or spinach leaves.

Preparation time: 30 minutes.

Servings: 4 people.

Miso soup with mushrooms and tofu

Ingredients:

- 4 cups of vegetable broth

- 1 cup of water

- 1/2 cup dried shiitake mushrooms

- 1/2 cup firm tofu cut into cubes

- 2 tablespoons of white miso paste

- 1 green onion chopped

- 1 tablespoon sesame oil

- 1 clove of garlic, minced

- 1 tablespoon grated ginger

- 1 tablespoon soy sauce

- 1 tablespoon of rice vinegar

- 1 tablespoon of brown sugar

- 1/4 cup chopped cilantro

• 2 tablespoons toasted sesame seeds

Instructions:

1) In a bowl, cover the shiitake mushrooms with hot water and let them soak for 10-15 minutes.

2) In a large pot, heat the sesame oil over medium heat. Add the green onion, garlic, and grated ginger. Cook for a few minutes until the green onion is soft.

3) Add the shiitake mushrooms (drain them first) and cook for a few minutes until golden.

4) Add the vegetable broth and water to the pot. Bring to a boil, then reduce the heat and simmer for about 10 minutes.

5) Add the cubed tofu and cook for another 5 minutes.

6) In a small bowl, mix the miso paste with some of the hot liquid from the soup until well combined. Add this mixture to the soup and stir well.

7) Add soy sauce, rice vinegar and brown sugar. Stir well to combine everything.

8) Serve the soup in bowls and decorate with chopped cilantro and toasted sesame seeds.

Preparation time: 30 minutes.

Servings: 4 people.

Chicken curry with broccoli and carrot

Ingredients:

• 4 boneless, skinless chicken breasts

• 1 tablespoon of vegetable oil

• 1 chopped onion

• 2 cloves of garlic, minced

- 1 tablespoon grated fresh ginger

- 2 tablespoons curry powder

- 1 tablespoon tomato paste

- 1 cup chicken broth

- 1 cup of coconut milk

- 1 head of broccoli cut into florets

- 2 carrots peeled and cut into slices

- Salt and pepper to taste

- Cooked rice to accompany

Instructions:

1) Preheat the oven to 200°C.

2) Cut the chicken into small cubes and season with salt and pepper to taste.

3) In a large skillet, heat the oil over medium heat. Add the chicken and cook for 6-7 minutes until golden brown on all sides.

4) Remove the chicken from the pan and set aside.

5) In the same pan, add the onion and cook for 3-4 minutes until golden. Then, add the garlic and grated ginger and cook for 1 more minute.

6) Add the curry powder and tomato paste and cook for 1 more minute.

7) Add the chicken broth and coconut milk and mix well. Then, add the broccoli and carrots and mix well.

8) Add the reserved chicken to the pan and mix well. Adjust salt and pepper to taste.

9) Transfer the pan to the oven and cook for 20-25 minutes until the vegetables are tender.

10) Serve hot with cooked rice.

Preparation time: approximately 30 minutes.

Cooking time: approximately 25 to 30 minutes.

Servings: 4 people.

Grilled tofu with carrot and cucumber salad

Ingredients:

- 400g firm tofu

- 2 tablespoons of olive oil

- 2 teaspoons of grated ginger

- 2 teaspoons minced garlic

- 2 teaspoons soy sauce

- 2 medium carrots, peeled and grated

- 2 small cucumbers, peeled and cut into thin strips

- 1/4 cup rice vinegar

- 1 tablespoon of honey

- 1 tablespoon sesame oil

- 1 tablespoon toasted sesame seeds

- Salt and pepper to taste

Instructions:

1) Cut the tofu into thin pieces and put them in a deep plate.

2) In a small bowl, mix the olive oil, grated ginger, minced garlic, and soy sauce. Pour the mixture over the tofu and make sure to coat all the pieces well.

3) Let the tofu marinate for 10-15 minutes.

4) Preheat grill or skillet over medium-high heat.

5) Meanwhile, in a large bowl, mix the grated carrots, thinly sliced cucumbers, rice vinegar, honey, and sesame oil.

6) Add salt and pepper to taste and mix well.

7) Place the marinated tofu on the hot grill or skillet and cook for 3-4 minutes on each side, or until golden brown and crispy.

8) Serve the grilled tofu with the carrot and cucumber salad and sprinkle toasted sesame seeds on top.

Preparation time: 30 minutes

Servings: 4 people.

Quinoa salad with avocado and tomato

Ingredients:

- 1 cup of quinoa

- 2 cups of water

- 2 medium tomatoes, diced

- 1 large avocado, peeled and cut into cubes

- 1/2 cup chopped red onion

- 1/4 cup chopped fresh cilantro

- 1/4 cup fresh lemon juice

- 2 tablespoons of olive oil

- Salt and pepper to taste

Instructions:

1) Rinse the quinoa with cold water in a fine strainer and let it drain.

2) Place the quinoa and 2 cups of water in a saucepan and bring to a boil over high heat. Reduce the heat to medium-low and cover the saucepan. Cook the

quinoa for 15-20 minutes or until it is tender, and the water has completely evaporated.

3) Meanwhile, prepare the salad ingredients. Mix tomatoes, avocado, red onion, and cilantro in a large bowl.

4) In a small bowl, mix the lemon juice, olive oil, salt, and pepper.

5) When the quinoa is ready, add it to the salad mixture and stir well.

6) Add the lemon and olive oil dressing and mix well.

7) Serve the quinoa salad with avocado and tomato on individual plates and enjoy.

Preparation time: 25 minutes.

Servings: 4 people.

Kale and potato soup

Ingredients:

- 1 large onion, chopped

- 2 cloves of garlic, minced

- 4 cups of chicken or vegetable broth

- 4 cups kale, chopped

- 2 large potatoes, peeled and cut into cubes

- 1 teaspoon dried thyme

- 1 teaspoon salt

- 1/2 teaspoon ground black pepper

- 2 tablespoons of olive oil

Instructions:

1) Heat the olive oil in a large pot over medium-high heat. Add the onion and garlic, and cook for 2-3 minutes, or until soft and fragrant.

2) Add the potatoes to the pot and cook for another 2-3 minutes, or until lightly browned.

3) Add the kale to the pot and mix well. Cook for 1-2 minutes, or until the kale softens slightly.

4) Add the chicken or vegetable broth to the pot, along with the thyme, salt, and pepper. Mix well.

5) Bring the soup to a boil, then reduce the heat to medium-low and simmer for 20-25 minutes, or until the potatoes are soft.

6) Once the potatoes are cooked, remove the pot from the heat and let it cool slightly.

7) Using a blender or food processor, blend the soup until smooth. If the soup is too thick, add a little more broth to thin it out.

8) Reheat the soup before serving, if necessary. It can be served with some crusty bread or crackers.

Preparation time: 15 minutes

Cooking time: 25 minutes

Servings: 4 people.

Grilled salmon with mango sauce

Ingredients:

- 4 salmon fillets of 150 g each

- 2 ripe mangoes

- 1 red onion

- 1 fresh red chili

- 1 lemon

- 1/4 cup chopped fresh cilantro

- Salt and ground black pepper

- Olive oil

Instructions:

1) Peel and chop the mangoes and red onion into small cubes. Finely chop the red chili and fresh cilantro. Mix all the ingredients in a bowl and squeeze the juice of half a lemon. Season with salt and pepper to taste and let it rest in the refrigerator.

2) Preheat the grill to medium-high heat. Season the salmon fillets with salt and pepper and brush them with olive oil.

3) Place the salmon fillets on the grill skin side down and cook for 4-5 minutes on each side, or until golden brown and cooked to desired doneness.

4) Serve the salmon fillets hot with the mango sauce on top. Serve with a side of rice, potatoes, or vegetables to taste.

Preparation time: 25 minutes.

Servings: 4 people.

Baked chicken with lemon and garlic

Ingredients:

- 4 chicken breasts

- 3 cloves of garlic, minced

- 1/4 cup lemon juice

- 2 tablespoons of olive oil

- 1 tablespoon dried oregano

- Salt and pepper to taste

• Lemon slices to decorate

Instructions:

1) Preheat the oven to 200°C.

2) In a small bowl, mix the garlic, lemon juice, olive oil and oregano.

3) Place the chicken breasts on a baking sheet and season with salt and pepper to taste.

4) Pour the lemon and garlic mixture over the chicken breasts, making sure they are well coated.

5) Bake for 25-30 minutes or until chicken is cooked through.

6) Serve hot and decorate with lemon slices.

Preparation time: 10 minutes

Cooking time: 25-30 minutes

Servings: 4 people.

Kale and lentil salad

Ingredients:

• 1/2 cup dried lentils

• 1 bunch of kale

• 1/2 red onion, chopped

• 1/2 cup grated carrot

• 1/2 cup crumbled feta cheese

• 1/4 cup olive oil

• 2 tablespoons apple cider vinegar

• 1 tablespoon of honey

• Salt and pepper to taste

Instructions:

1) Cook lentils according to package instructions and set aside.

2) Wash and dry the kale, remove the leaves from the stems and chop them into small pieces.

3) In a large bowl, combine the kale, red onion, shredded carrot, and crumbled feta cheese. Mix well.

4) In another bowl, whisk together the olive oil, apple cider vinegar, honey, salt, and pepper to make the dressing.

5) Add the cooked lentils to the salad and toss with the dressing.

6) Serve the salad immediately or refrigerate for at least 30 minutes before serving to allow the flavors to combine.

Preparation time: 20 minutes (more cooking time for the lentils if necessary).

Total time: 50 minutes (including cooling time in the refrigerator).

Servings: 4 people.

<u>Chicken tacos with coleslaw and cilantro</u>

Ingredients:

• 1 tablespoon olive oil

• 4 boneless, skinless chicken breasts

• 2 tablespoons of fresh lemon juice

• 1 tablespoon of ground cumin

• 1 tablespoon chili powder

• 1 tablespoon garlic powder

• 1/2 teaspoon salt

- 1/2 teaspoon black pepper

- 8 corn or flour tortillas

- 1/2 head of red cabbage, grated

- 1/2 cup chopped fresh cilantro

- 1/4 cup chopped red onion

- 1/4 cup sour cream (optional)

Instructions:

1) Preheat the oven to 200°C. In a large skillet, heat the olive oil over medium-high heat.

2) Meanwhile, in a medium bowl, mix the lemon juice, cumin, chili powder, garlic powder, salt, and pepper.

3) Cut the chicken into strips and add to the spice mixture, making sure it is well coated.

4) Place the chicken strips in the hot pan and cook for 5-7 minutes on each side, until golden brown and cooked through.

5) Meanwhile, heat the tortillas in a frying pan or in the microwave.

6) In a large bowl, mix the shredded cabbage, cilantro and red onion.

7) To assemble the tacos, place a portion of chicken in the center of each hot tortilla. Top with a spoonful of the cilantro coleslaw and a little sour cream if desired.

8) Serve immediately and enjoy.

Preparation time: 25 minutes

Servings: 4 people.

Salmon burgers with avocado and yogurt sauce

Ingredients:

• 500 grams of fresh salmon without skin or bones

• 1 ripe avocado

• 1/4 cup breadcrumbs

• 1 egg

• 1/4 teaspoon salt

• 1/4 teaspoon ground black pepper

• 2 tablespoons of olive oil

• 4 hamburger buns

• 1 cup chopped lettuce

• 1 ripe tomato sliced

For the yogurt sauce:

• 1/2 cup plain Greek yogurt

• 1 tablespoon lemon juice

• 1 clove of garlic, minced

• 1/4 teaspoon salt

• 1/4 teaspoon ground black pepper

Instructions:

1) Preheat the oven to 180°C.

2) Cut the salmon into pieces and place in a food processor. Process until finely chopped.

3) Add the avocado, breadcrumbs, egg, salt, and pepper. Process again until the mixture is homogeneous.

4) Divide the salmon mixture into 4 portions and form into burgers.

5) Heat the olive oil in a large skillet over medium-high heat. Add the salmon burgers and cook for 3-4 minutes on each side or until golden brown.

6) Transfer the salmon burgers to a baking sheet and bake for 8-10 minutes or until cooked.

7) To make the yogurt sauce, mix the yogurt, lemon juice, garlic, salt, and pepper in a small bowl.

8) Place a salmon burger on each burger bun and cover with lettuce, tomato, and yogurt sauce. Serve and enjoy!

Preparation time: 30 minutes.

Cooking time: 15 minutes.

Servings: 4 people.

Pumpkin and ginger soup

Ingredients:

• 1 kg of pumpkin

• 1 chopped onion

• 2 cloves of garlic, minced

• 1 piece of fresh ginger about 3 cm, peeled and finely chopped

• 4 cups of vegetable broth

• 1/2 cup coconut milk

• Salt and ground black pepper

• Olive oil

• Pumpkin seeds to decorate (optional)

Instructions:

1) Peel and cut the pumpkin into small pieces. Reserve.

2) Heat a tablespoon of olive oil in a large pot over medium heat. Add the onion and garlic and cook for a few minutes until soft.

3) Add the chopped ginger and pumpkin pieces to the pot. Cook for a few more minutes.

4) Add the vegetable broth to the pot. Bring to a boil, reduce heat to medium-low, and simmer until squash is tender.

5) Remove the soup from the heat and use a hand blender to puree until smooth.

6) Add the coconut milk and mix well.

7) Return the soup to the pot and heat over medium-low heat.

8) Adjust the flavor with salt and pepper.

9) Serve hot and decorate with pumpkin seeds if you wish.

Preparation time: 15 minutes.

Cooking time: 30-40 minutes.

Servings: 4 people.

Lentil salad with avocado and cucumber

Ingredients:

- 1 cup of cooked lentils

- 1 ripe avocado, cut into cubes

- 1 medium cucumber, peeled and sliced

- 1 medium tomato, cut into cubes

- 1/4 red onion, finely chopped

- Juice of 1 lemon

- 2 tablespoons of olive oil

• Salt and pepper to taste

• Fresh coriander leaves (optional, to decorate)

Instructions:

1) In a large bowl, combine the cooked lentils, avocado, cucumber, tomato and red onion.

2) In another small bowl, mix the lemon juice, olive oil, salt, and pepper. Beat well to emulsify the ingredients.

3) Pour the dressing mixture over the lentil salad and stir gently to combine all the ingredients.

4) Garnish with fresh cilantro leaves, if desired.

5) Serve the lentil salad immediately or refrigerate it for a while to serve cold.

Preparation time: Approximately 15 minutes.

Servings: 4 people.

Baked salmon with honey mustard crust

Ingredients:

• 4 salmon fillets (150-200 grams each)

• 2 tablespoons Dijon mustard

• 2 tablespoons of honey

• 2 tablespoons of olive oil

• Juice of 1 lemon

• Salt and pepper to taste

• Chopped fresh parsley (optional, to decorate)

Instructions:

1) Preheat the oven to 200°C (400°F) and line a baking sheet with aluminum foil or baking paper.

2) In a small bowl, mix Dijon mustard, honey, olive oil, lemon juice, salt, and pepper. Mix all the ingredients well until you obtain a homogeneous sauce.

3) Place the salmon fillets on the prepared baking sheet and pour the honey mustard sauce over each one, making sure to cover them completely.

4) Bake the salmon for approximately 12-15 minutes, or until cooked and flakes easily with a fork.

5) Remove the salmon from the oven and decorate with fresh chopped parsley, if desired.

6) Serve the baked salmon with a hot honey mustard crust and accompany it with a side dish of your choice, such as steamed vegetables or salad.

Preparation time: Approximately 20 minutes.

Servings: 4 people.

Grilled chicken with yogurt and cucumber sauce

Ingredients:

• 4 boneless, skinless chicken breasts

• 1/2 cup of natural unsweetened yogurt

• 1/2 medium cucumber, peeled and grated

• 2 cloves of garlic, minced

• Juice of 1 lemon

• 2 tablespoons of olive oil

• 1 teaspoon ground cumin

• Salt and pepper to taste

• Fresh mint leaves (optional, to decorate)

Instructions:

1) In a bowl, mix the yogurt, grated cucumber, garlic, lemon juice, olive oil, cumin, salt, and pepper. Mix all the ingredients well to obtain the yogurt and cucumber sauce. Reserve in the refrigerator.

2) Preheat the grill to medium-high heat.

3) Season the chicken breasts with salt and pepper to taste.

4) Place the chicken breasts on the hot grill and cook for approximately 6-8 minutes on each side, or until cooked through and reach an internal temperature of 75°C (165°F).

5) Remove the chicken from the grill and let it rest for a few minutes.

6) Serve the grilled chicken breasts with the yogurt and cucumber sauce on top. You can decorate with fresh mint leaves if you wish.

7) Accompany the chicken with a garnish of your choice, such as green salad or brown rice.

Preparation time: Approximately 25 minutes.

Servings: 4 people.

Quinoa salad with tomato and cilantro

Ingredients:

- 1 cup of quinoa

- 2 cups of water

- 2 medium tomatoes, diced

- 1/2 red onion, finely chopped

- 1 bunch of fresh cilantros, chopped

- Juice of 1 lemon

- 2 tablespoons of olive oil

• Salt and pepper to taste

• Lettuce leaves (optional, to serve)

Instructions:

1) Rinse the quinoa under cold water to remove any bitter residue. Then, place it in a saucepan with 2 cups of water and bring to a boil.

2) Reduce the heat to low, cover the saucepan, and cook the quinoa for about 15 minutes, or until it is tender and has absorbed all the liquid. Remove from heat and let sit for a few minutes.

3) In a large bowl, combine the cooked quinoa, diced tomatoes, chopped red onion, and fresh cilantro.

4) In another small bowl, mix the lemon juice, olive oil, salt, and pepper. Blend well to emulsify the ingredients and then pour the mixture over the quinoa salad. Mix gently to combine all ingredients.

5) Optionally, you can serve the quinoa salad on lettuce leaves for a more attractive presentation.

6) Serve the Quinoa Salad with Tomato and Cilantro immediately or refrigerate it for a while to serve cold.

Preparation time: Approximately 25 minutes.

Servings: 4 people.

Fish soup with vegetables

Ingredients:

• 500 grams of white fish fillets (such as hake or sole), cut into pieces

• 1 chopped onion

• 2 carrots, cut into slices

• 2 stalks of celery, cut into pieces

- 1 red pepper, cut into pieces

- 2 cloves of garlic, minced

- 1 can (400 grams) of peeled tomatoes, chopped

- 4 cups of fish broth or vegetable broth

- 1 teaspoon turmeric powder

- 1 teaspoon ground cumin

- Salt and pepper to taste

- Olive oil for cooking

- Fresh parsley leaves (optional, to decorate)

Instructions:

1) In a large pot, heat some olive oil over medium heat. Add the onion, carrots, celery, red pepper, and garlic. Cook until the vegetables are tender, about 5 minutes.

2) Add the chopped tomatoes to the pot and cook for another 2 minutes.

3) Add the fish broth or vegetable broth to the pot. Then, add the turmeric, cumin, salt, and pepper. Mix well.

4) Bring the soup to a boil and reduce the heat to low. Simmer for about 15 minutes to let the flavors blend.

5) Add the fish pieces to the pot and cook for about 5 minutes, or until the fish is cooked and flakes easily.

6) Remove the pot from the heat and let the soup sit for a few minutes.

7) Serve the fish soup with vegetables hot and decorate with fresh parsley leaves if you wish.

Preparation time: Approximately 30 minutes.

Servings: 4 people.

Chickpea curry with spinach and tomato

Ingredients:

• 2 cans (400 grams each) of chickpeas, rinsed and drained

• 2 cups of fresh spinach

• 1 chopped onion

• 2 cloves of garlic, minced

• 1 red pepper, cut into pieces

• 1 can (400 grams) of peeled tomatoes, chopped

• 1 can (400 ml) of coconut milk

• 2 tablespoons curry paste (you can adjust the amount according to your spiciness preference)

• 1 teaspoon turmeric powder

• 1 teaspoon ground cumin

• Salt and pepper to taste

• Olive oil for cooking

• Brown rice or cooked quinoa (optional, to serve)

Instructions:

1) In a large pot, heat some olive oil over medium heat. Add the onion and garlic, and cook until golden and fragrant, about 5 minutes.

2) Add the red pepper to the pot and cook for another 2 minutes.

3) Add the curry paste, turmeric, and cumin to the pot, and stir to mix the spices with the vegetables.

4) Add the chopped tomatoes and cook for a few more minutes.

5) Add the drained chickpeas to the pot, followed by the coconut milk. Mix all the ingredients well and bring to a boil.

6) Reduce the heat to low and let the curry cook for about 15-20 minutes, so that the flavors blend and the chickpeas heat through.

7) Add the fresh spinach to the pot and cook until wilted, about 5 minutes.

8) Taste the curry and adjust the seasoning with salt and pepper as needed.

9) Serve the chickpea curry with spinach and tomato hot, accompanied by brown rice or cooked quinoa if you wish.

Preparation time: Approximately 40 minutes.

Servings: 4 people.

Chicken curry with coconut milk and peppers

Ingredients:

• 500 grams of chicken breasts, cut into pieces

• 1 chopped onion

• 2 cloves of garlic, minced

• 1 red pepper, cut into pieces

• 1 green pepper, cut into pieces

• 1 can (400 ml) of coconut milk

• 2 tablespoons curry paste

• 1 teaspoon turmeric powder

• 1 teaspoon ground cumin

• Salt and pepper to taste

• Olive oil for cooking

• Fresh coriander leaves (optional, to decorate)

• Brown rice or cooked quinoa (optional, to serve)

Instructions:

1) In a large skillet, heat some olive oil over medium heat. Add the onion and garlic, and cook until golden and fragrant, about 5 minutes.

2) Add the chicken pieces to the pan and cook until golden brown on all sides.

3) Add the cut peppers to the pan and cook for a few more minutes.

4) In a separate bowl, mix the curry paste, turmeric and cumin. Add this mixture to the pan and stir so that the spices are distributed throughout the preparation.

5) Pour the coconut milk into the pan and mix all the ingredients well. Bring the mixture to a boil and then reduce the heat to medium-low.

6) Cook the chicken curry for about 15-20 minutes, or until the chicken is cooked through and tender. Stir occasionally to make sure it doesn't stick to the bottom of the pan.

7) Taste the curry and adjust the seasoning with salt and pepper as needed.

8) Serve the chicken curry with coconut milk and peppers hot, accompanied by brown rice or cooked quinoa if you wish. Garnish with fresh cilantro leaves if you prefer.

Preparation time: Approximately 30 minutes.

Servings: 4 people.

Grilled tofu with peanut sauce

Ingredients:

• 400 grams of firm tofu, cut into fillets

• 1/4 cup low sodium soy sauce

• 2 tablespoons sesame oil

• 2 tablespoons of natural peanut sauce

- 2 tablespoons of lemon juice

- 1 tablespoon honey or agave syrup (optional, to sweeten)

- 2 cloves of garlic, minced

- 1 teaspoon grated fresh ginger

- 2 chives, chopped

- Toasted sesame seeds (optional, to decorate)

- Fresh coriander leaves (optional, to decorate)

Instructions:

1) In a small bowl, whisk together the soy sauce, sesame oil, peanut sauce, lemon juice, minced garlic, grated ginger, and honey or agave syrup (if desired). This mixture will be the marinade and sauce for the tofu.

2) Place the tofu fillets in a shallow bowl and pour the marinade over them. Make sure the fillets are well coated with the marinade. Marinate for at least 15 minutes to absorb the flavors.

3) Heat a grill or skillet over medium-high heat. Remove the tofu fillets from the marinade and reserve the marinade for the sauce.

4) Cook the tofu fillets on the hot grill or pan for about 4-5 minutes on each side, or until golden brown and crispy.

5) While the tofu is cooking, you can prepare the sauce. In a small skillet, pour the reserved marinade and heat over medium-low heat. Cook the sauce for a few minutes, stirring occasionally, until it thickens slightly.

6) Serve the grilled tofu fillets with the hot peanut sauce. Sprinkle toasted sesame seeds and fresh coriander leaves on top if desired.

Preparation time: Approximately 30 minutes (including marinating time).

Servings: 4 people

Spinach salad with strawberries and walnuts

Ingredients:

- 8 cups of fresh spinach

- 1 cup strawberries, washed and sliced

- 1/2 cup chopped walnuts

- 1/4 cup crumbled feta cheese (optional)

- 2 tablespoons of olive oil

- 2 tablespoons balsamic vinegar

- 1 tablespoon honey or agave syrup (optional, to sweeten)

- Salt and pepper to taste

Instructions:

1) In a large bowl, combine the spinach, sliced strawberries, chopped walnuts, and crumbled feta cheese (if desired).

2) In another smaller container, mix the olive oil, balsamic vinegar, and honey or agave syrup (if desired) to make the dressing.

3) Pour the dressing over the salad and toss gently to make sure all the ingredients are well coated.

4) Season the salad with salt and pepper to taste.

5) Serve the spinach salad with strawberries and walnuts immediately and enjoy its freshness and flavor.

Preparation time: Approximately 10 minutes.

Servings: 4 people

Baked salmon with dill sauce

Ingredients:

• 4 salmon fillets (approximately 150 grams each)

• Salt and pepper to taste

• 2 tablespoons of olive oil

• 2 tablespoons chopped fresh dill

For the dill sauce:

• 1 cup of Greek yogurt

• 2 tablespoons chopped fresh dill

• 1 clove of garlic, minced

• Juice of half a lemon

• Salt and pepper to taste

Instructions:

1) Preheat the oven to 200°C (400°F) and prepare a baking sheet lined with aluminum foil.

2) Wash the salmon fillets and dry them with kitchen paper. Place them on the baking sheet and season with salt and pepper to taste.

3) In a separate bowl, mix the olive oil and chopped fresh dill. Pour this mixture over the salmon fillets, making sure to cover them completely.

4) Bake the salmon in the preheated oven for about 15-18 minutes, or until cooked and flakes easily with a fork.

5) While the salmon is baking, prepare the dill sauce. In a bowl, mix together the Greek yogurt, chopped fresh dill, minced garlic, and lemon juice. Stir all the ingredients well until you obtain a homogeneous sauce. Season with salt and pepper to taste.

6) Once the salmon is ready, serve it hot accompanied by the dill sauce. You can add a side of salad or vegetables on the side if you wish.

Preparation time: 25 minutes

Servings: 4 people

Chickpea and cucumber salad

Ingredients:

- 2 cups of cooked chickpeas

- 1 large cucumber, cut into cubes

- 1 large tomato, cut into cubes

- 1/2 red onion, finely chopped

- 1 red pepper, cut into cubes

- 1/4 cup pitted black olives, sliced

- 1/4 cup chopped fresh parsley

- 2 tablespoons of olive oil

- Juice of 1 lemon

- Salt and pepper to taste

Instructions:

1) In a large bowl, combine the cooked chickpeas, cucumber, tomato, red onion, red pepper, black olives and chopped fresh parsley.

2) In another small bowl, mix the olive oil, lemon juice, salt, and pepper. Stir well to combine the ingredients and form the dressing.

3) Pour the dressing over the chickpea and cucumber salad and toss gently to make sure all the ingredients are well coated.

4) Let the salad sit in the refrigerator for at least 30 minutes before serving, so the flavors can blend.

5) Serve the Anti-Inflammatory Chickpea and Cucumber Salad cold and enjoy it as a main dish or as a side dish.

Preparation time: 15 minutes

Servings: 4 people

Chicken tacos with mango and cilantro salsa

Ingredients:

• 4 corn or wheat flour tortillas

• 2 boneless, skinless chicken breasts, cut into strips

• 1 ripe mango, peeled and cut into cubes

• 1/2 red onion, chopped

• 1/4 cup chopped fresh cilantro

• Juice of 1 lime

• 2 tablespoons of olive oil

• Salt and pepper to taste

Instructions:

1) In a large skillet, heat the olive oil over medium-high heat. Add the chicken strips and season with salt and pepper to taste. Cook the chicken for approximately 8-10 minutes, or until cooked through and golden brown. Remove from heat and reserve.

2) In a bowl, mix the mango cubes, chopped red onion, chopped fresh cilantro and lime juice. Stir well to combine all the ingredients and form the mango and cilantro sauce. Season with salt and pepper to taste.

3) Heat the tortillas in a skillet or in the microwave until hot and pliable.

4) Fill each tortilla with the cooked chicken strips and add a tablespoon of the mango and cilantro sauce on top.

5) Fold the tortillas to form tacos and serve hot.

Preparation time: 25 minutes

Servings: 4 people

Tomato and pepper soup

Ingredients:

- 4 large tomatoes, peeled and cut into pieces

- 2 large red peppers, roasted and peeled

- 1 large onion, chopped

- 2 cloves of garlic, minced

- 4 cups of vegetable broth

- 2 tablespoons of olive oil

- 1 teaspoon ground cumin

- 1 teaspoon paprika

- Salt and pepper to taste

- Fresh basil leaves to decorate (optional)

Instructions:

1) In a large pot, heat the olive oil over medium heat. Add the chopped onion and garlic and cook until tender and lightly browned.

2) Add the chopped tomatoes and roasted red peppers to the pot. Cook for a few minutes until the ingredients are well mixed and softened.

3) Add the vegetable broth to the pot and bring the mixture to a boil. Reduce the heat and let the soup simmer for about 15-20 minutes to allow the flavors to blend.

4) Remove the pot from the heat and let the soup cool slightly. Then, use a blender or hand blender to puree the soup until smooth and creamy. If you prefer a coarser texture, you can leave some pieces uncrushed.

5) Return the soup to the pot and heat over medium heat. Add the ground cumin, paprika, salt and pepper to taste. Stir well to incorporate the seasonings.

6) Once the soup is hot, serve in individual bowls and garnish with fresh basil leaves if desired.

Preparation time: 30 minutes

Servings: 4 people

Quinoa salad with avocado and orange

Ingredients:

- 1 cup quinoa, rinsed

- 2 cups of water

- 2 ripe avocados, cut into cubes

- 2 oranges, peeled and separated into segments

- 1/2 red onion, finely chopped

- 1/4 cup chopped fresh cilantro

- Juice of 1 lemon

- 2 tablespoons of olive oil

- Salt and pepper to taste

Instructions:

1) In a medium pot, bring the water to a boil. Add the quinoa and reduce the heat to low. Cook the quinoa, covered, for about 15 minutes, or until it is

tender and has absorbed all the liquid. Remove from heat and let sit, covered, for another 5 minutes. Then, uncover and let cool.

2) In a large bowl, combine the cooked quinoa, avocado cubes, orange segments, chopped red onion, and chopped fresh cilantro.

3) In another small bowl, mix the lemon juice, olive oil, salt, and pepper. Stir well to combine the ingredients and form the dressing.

4) Pour the dressing over the quinoa salad and toss gently to make sure all the ingredients are well coated.

5) Let the salad sit in the refrigerator for at least 30 minutes before serving, so the flavors can blend, and the salad is fresh.

6) Serve the Anti-Inflammatory Orange Avocado Quinoa Salad cold as a main dish or as a side dish.

Preparation time: 20 minutes

Servings: 4 people

Grilled chicken with cabbage and carrot salad

Ingredients:

- 4 boneless, skinless chicken breasts

- Salt and pepper to taste

- 2 tablespoons of olive oil

For the cabbage and carrot salad:

- 3 cups of shredded cabbage

- 2 large carrots, grated

- 1/4 cup Greek yogurt

- 2 tablespoons apple cider vinegar

- 1 tablespoon Dijon mustard

• 1 teaspoon honey (optional)

• Salt and pepper to taste

Instructions:

1) Preheat the grill to medium-high heat.

2) Season the chicken breasts with salt and pepper to taste. Drizzle the olive oil over the chicken so it doesn't stick to the grill.

3) Place the chicken breasts on the hot grill and cook for approximately 6-8 minutes on each side, or until cooked through and reach an internal temperature of 75°C (165°F). Cooking time may vary depending on the thickness of the chicken breasts.

4) While the chicken is cooking, prepare the cabbage and carrot salad. In a large bowl, combine the shredded cabbage and carrots.

5) In another small bowl, mix the greek yogurt, apple cider vinegar, dijon mustard, honey (if desired), salt and pepper. Stir well to combine the ingredients and form the dressing.

6) Pour the dressing over the shredded cabbage and carrots. Mix well to make sure all ingredients are coated.

7) Once the chicken is ready, remove it from the grill and let it rest for a few minutes. Then cut it into slices or pieces.

8) Serve the Grilled Chicken along with the anti-inflammatory cabbage and carrot salad. You can add an additional vegetable garnish if you wish.

Preparation time: 30 minutes

Servings: 4 people

Grilled salmon with fresh herbs

Ingredients:

- 4 salmon fillets (approximately 150 g each)

- Salt and pepper to taste

- 2 tablespoons of olive oil

- 2 tablespoons of lemon juice

- 2 tablespoons chopped fresh parsley

- 2 tablespoons chopped fresh dill

- 2 tablespoons chopped fresh basil

- Lemon slices to decorate (optional)

Instructions:

1) Preheat the grill to medium-high heat.

2) Season the salmon fillets with salt and pepper to taste.

3) In a small bowl, mix the olive oil, lemon juice, chopped parsley, chopped dill and basil. Stir well to combine the herbs and form the dressing.

4) Place the salmon fillets on the hot grill and cook for about 4-6 minutes on each side, or until cooked through and flake easily with a fork.

5) During the last few minutes of cooking, brush the salmon fillets with the fresh herb dressing, turning once to coat both sides. Reserve some dressing to serve.

6) Remove the salmon from the grill and place it on a plate. Drizzle with remaining fresh herb dressing.

7) Garnish with lemon slices, if desired, and serve the Grilled Salmon with fresh anti-inflammatory herbs hot.

Preparation time: 15 minutes

Servings: 4 people

Kale salad with turmeric and ginger

Ingredients:

• 1 bunch kale, chopped into small pieces

• 2 tablespoons of olive oil

• 1 teaspoon turmeric powder

• 1 teaspoon grated fresh ginger

• Juice of 1 lemon

• 1/4 cup sunflower seeds

• 1/4 cup raisins

• Salt and pepper to taste

Instructions:

1) In a large bowl, place the chopped kale.

2) In a small skillet, heat the olive oil over medium heat. Add turmeric powder and grated ginger. Cook for a few minutes to release the aromas.

3) Pour the olive oil, turmeric, and ginger mixture over the kale. Add the lemon juice and season with salt and pepper to taste.

4) With clean hands, gently massage the kale for a few minutes to soften it and allow the flavors to blend.

5) Add the sunflower seeds and raisins to the salad. Mix well to distribute the ingredients.

6) Let the salad sit for a few minutes so that the flavors intensify, and the ingredients combine.

7) Serve Anti-Inflammatory Ginger Turmeric Kale Salad as a side or main dish.

Preparation time: 15 minutes

Servings: 4 people

Pork chops with applesauce and cinnamon

Ingredients:

• 4 pork chops

• Salt and pepper to taste

• 2 tablespoons of olive oil

• For the applesauce and cinnamon:

• 4 apples, peeled, cored, and cut into pieces

• 1 teaspoon cinnamon powder

• 1 tablespoon lemon juice

• 2 tablespoons of honey (optional)

• 1/4 cup of water

Instructions:

1) Preheat the oven to 200°C (400°F).

2) Season the pork chops with salt and pepper to taste.

3) Heat the olive oil in a large skillet over medium-high heat. Add the pork chops and cook for 3-4 minutes on each side, or until golden brown.

4) Transfer the pork chops to a baking sheet and place in the preheated oven. Cook for approximately 10-15 minutes, or until the chops are cooked through and reach an internal temperature of 70°C (160°F).

5) Meanwhile, prepare the apple and cinnamon puree. In a medium pot, place the apple pieces, cinnamon powder, lemon juice, honey (if desired) and water. Cook over medium heat for approximately 15-20 minutes, or until the apples are tender and can be mashed easily.

6) Remove the pot from the heat and use a fork or food processor to mash the apples until smooth and creamy.

7) Serve the pork chops along with the anti-inflammatory applesauce and cinnamon. You can add a side of steamed vegetables or a fresh salad if you wish.

Preparation time: 40 minutes

Servings: 4 people

Lentil stew with spices

Ingredients:

- 1 cup of lentils

- 2 tablespoons of olive oil

- 1 medium onion, chopped

- 2 carrots, sliced

- 2 stalks of celery, sliced

- 3 cloves of garlic, minced

- 1 teaspoon ground cumin

- 1 teaspoon turmeric powder

- 1/2 teaspoon paprika

- 1 can (400 g) of crushed tomatoes

- 4 cups of vegetable broth

- Salt and pepper to taste

- Fresh coriander leaves to decorate (optional)

Instructions:

1) Rinse the lentils with cold water and drain them.

2) In a large pot, heat the olive oil over medium heat. Add the onion, carrots, and celery and cook until tender, about 5 minutes.

3) Add the garlic, cumin, turmeric and paprika to the pot. Cook for 1 minute, stirring constantly so the spices are mixed well.

4) Add the crushed tomatoes and lentils to the pot. Mix everything together.

5) Pour the vegetable broth into the pot and bring the mixture to a boil. Reduce the heat to medium-low, cover the pot, and let it simmer for about 30 minutes or until the lentils are tender.

6) If necessary, add more vegetable broth during cooking if the stew becomes too thick.

7) Once the lentils are cooked, season the stew with salt and pepper to taste.

8) Serve the lentil stew hot and decorate with fresh cilantro leaves if you wish.

Preparation time: Approximately 45 minutes.

Servings: 4 people

Brown rice with mushrooms and garlic

Ingredients:

• 1 cup of brown rice

• 2 cups of vegetable broth

• 2 tablespoons of olive oil

• 4 cloves of garlic, minced

• 250 g mushrooms (such as button mushrooms), sliced

• 1 medium onion, chopped

• 1 red pepper, diced

• 1 teaspoon dried thyme

• 1 teaspoon dried rosemary

• Salt and pepper to taste

• Chopped fresh parsley to decorate (optional)

Instructions:

1) Rinse the brown rice with cold water and drain.

2) In a medium pot, bring the vegetable broth to a boil and then add the brown rice. Reduce heat to low, cover pot, and cook rice for about 30 minutes or according to package directions, until tender and broth has been absorbed. Remove from heat and let sit, covered, for 5 minutes.

3) While the rice is cooking, heat the olive oil in a large skillet over medium heat. Add the minced garlic and cook for 1 minute until fragrant.

4) Add the mushrooms to the pan and cook until they are tender and have released their juices, about 5 minutes.

5) Add the onion and red pepper to the skillet and cook until tender, about 5 minutes more.

6) Add the thyme and rosemary to the pan and mix everything together. Cook for 1 more minute.

7) Add the cooked rice to the pan with the sautéed ingredients. Mix well to combine all the flavors.

8) Season with salt and pepper to taste.

9) If desired, garnish brown rice with fresh chopped parsley before serving.

Preparation time: Approximately 40 minutes.

Servings: 4 people

Turkey burgers with spices and avocado

Ingredients:

• 500 g of ground turkey

• 1 ripe avocado, peeled and pitted

- 1 small onion, finely chopped

- 2 cloves of garlic, minced

- 1 teaspoon ground cumin

- 1 teaspoon paprika

- 1/2 teaspoon turmeric powder

- Salt and pepper to taste

- Olive oil for cooking

- Whole wheat or gluten-free rolls to serve

- Lettuce leaves and tomato slices to accompany

Instructions:

1) In a large bowl, combine the ground turkey, chopped onion, garlic, cumin, paprika, turmeric, salt, and pepper. Mix all ingredients well until well combined.

2) Divide the mixture into 4 equal parts and form patties with your hands. Make sure the burgers are a uniform thickness, so they cook evenly.

3) Heat a large skillet over medium-high heat and add a little olive oil.

4) Place the burgers on the hot skillet and cook for about 4-5 minutes on each side, or until golden brown and cooked through.

5) Meanwhile, mash the ripe avocado with a fork in a small bowl until smooth. Season with salt and pepper to taste.

6) Once the burgers are cooked, remove them from the heat and let them rest for a few minutes.

7) To assemble the burgers, place a turkey burger on a whole wheat or gluten-free bun. Spread a tablespoon of mashed avocado on the burger and add lettuce leaves and tomato slices.

8) Serve the turkey burgers with spices and avocado accompanied by a salad or steamed vegetables, if desired.

Preparation time: Approximately 30 minutes.

Servings: 4 people

Chickpea and spinach curry

Ingredients:

• 2 tablespoons of olive oil

• 1 medium onion, chopped

• 3 cloves of garlic, minced

• 1 tablespoon grated fresh ginger

• 2 tablespoons curry paste (you can adjust the amount according to your spiciness preference)

• 1 teaspoon turmeric powder

• 1 teaspoon ground cumin

• 1 can (400 g) of crushed tomatoes

• 1 can (400 ml) of coconut milk

• 2 cups of cooked chickpeas (can be canned)

• 4 cups of fresh spinach

• Salt to taste

• Chopped fresh cilantro to decorate (optional)

• Brown rice or cooked quinoa to serve

Instructions:

1) In a large pot, heat the olive oil over medium heat. Add the onion and cook until tender and translucent, about 5 minutes.

2) Add the garlic and grated ginger to the pot. Cook for 1 more minute, stirring constantly.

3) Add the curry paste, turmeric, and cumin to the pot. Cook for 1-2 minutes so the spices mix well.

4) Pour the crushed tomatoes into the pot and mix everything together. Cook for another 2 minutes.

5) Add the coconut milk to the pot and mix all the ingredients well.

6) Add the cooked chickpeas to the pot and cook over low heat for about 10 minutes so that the flavors integrate.

7) Add the fresh spinach to the pot and cook until wilted, about 3-4 minutes.

8) Season with salt to taste.

9) Serve the chickpea and spinach curry hot over brown rice or cooked quinoa.

10) Optionally, decorate with fresh chopped cilantro before serving.

Preparation time: Approximately 30 minutes.

Servings: 4 people

Avocado toast with egg and tomato

Ingredients:

- 4 slices of whole wheat or gluten-free bread

- 2 ripe avocados

- 4 eggs

- 2 medium tomatoes, sliced

- Juice of half a lemon

- Olive oil

- Salt and pepper to taste

- Chopped fresh cilantro to decorate (optional)

Instructions:

1) Toast the slices of whole wheat or gluten-free bread until crispy.

2) Meanwhile, peel and pit the avocados. Place the flesh of the avocados in a bowl and mash it with a fork until smooth.

3) Squeeze the juice of half a lemon over the avocado and mix well. Season with salt and pepper to taste.

4) In a large skillet, heat some olive oil over medium heat. Crack the eggs and place them in the pan. Cook eggs to your liking, whether scrambled, fried, or poached.

5) Spread a generous amount of mashed avocado on each slice of toast.

6) Place tomato slices on top of the mashed avocado on each toast.

7) Once the eggs are cooked, place one egg on each piece of toast.

8) Season the eggs with salt and pepper to taste.

9) Garnish with fresh chopped cilantro, if desired.

10) Serve the avocado toast with egg and tomato immediately.

Preparation time: Approximately 15 minutes.

Servings: 4 people

Baked salmon with honey mustard sauce

Ingredients:

- 4 salmon fillets (approximately 150 g each)

- 3 tablespoons Dijon mustard

- 2 tablespoons of honey

- 2 tablespoons of lemon juice

- 2 tablespoons of olive oil

- Salt and pepper to taste

• Lemon slices and fresh dill to decorate (optional)

Instructions:

1) Preheat the oven to 200°C.

2) In a small bowl, mix Dijon mustard, honey, lemon juice and olive oil. Mix well until you obtain a homogeneous sauce.

3) Place the salmon fillets on a baking sheet lined with aluminum foil or baking paper.

4) Season the salmon fillets with salt and pepper to taste.

5) Pour the honey mustard sauce over the salmon fillets, making sure to coat them evenly.

6) Bake the salmon for approximately 15-20 minutes, or until cooked and flakes easily with a fork. Cooking time may vary depending on the thickness of the fillets.

7) Remove the salmon from the oven and let it rest for a few minutes before serving.

8) Garnish with lemon slices and fresh dill, if desired.

9) Serve the baked salmon with honey mustard sauce along with a side of steamed vegetables or a fresh salad.

Preparation time: Approximately 25 minutes.

Servings: 4 people

Lentil soup with spinach and carrot

Ingredients:

• 1 cup of dried lentils

• 1 medium onion, chopped

• 2 large carrots, cut into cubes

- 2 bay leaves

- 3 cloves of garlic, minced

- 4 cups of vegetable broth

- 2 cups fresh spinach, washed and chopped

- 1 teaspoon turmeric powder

- 1 teaspoon ground cumin

- Salt and pepper to taste

- Olive oil for cooking

- Chopped fresh parsley to decorate (optional)

- Whole wheat or gluten-free bread to serve

Instructions:

1) Rinse the dried lentils with cold water and drain.

2) In a large pot, heat some olive oil over medium heat. Add the onion and carrots, and cook until tender, about 5 minutes.

3) Add the minced garlic, turmeric powder, and ground cumin to the pot. Cook for 1 more minute, stirring constantly to release the aromas of the spices.

4) Add the drained lentils and bay leaves to the pot. Mix all ingredients well.

5) Pour the vegetable broth into the pot and bring the mixture to a boil.

6) Reduce the heat to medium-low, cover the pot and simmer for about 25-30 minutes, or until the lentils are tender.

7) Add the fresh spinach to the pot and cook for 3-4 more minutes, or until the spinach wilts.

8) Season the soup with salt and pepper to taste.

9) Remove the bay leaves before serving.

10) Garnish with fresh chopped parsley, if desired.

11) Serve the lentil soup with spinach and carrot hot along with slices of whole wheat or gluten-free bread.

Preparation time: Approximately 40 minutes.

Servings: 4 people

Spinach, strawberry, and walnut salad

Ingredients:

- 8 cups of fresh spinach

- 2 cups strawberries, sliced

- 1/2 cup walnuts, chopped

- 1/4 cup crumbled feta cheese (optional)

- 2 tablespoons balsamic vinegar

- 2 tablespoons extra virgin olive oil

- 1 tablespoon of honey

- Salt and pepper to taste

Instructions:

1) In a large bowl, place the fresh spinach.

2) Add the sliced strawberries and chopped walnuts to the bowl.

3) If you wish, add the crumbled feta cheese to the salad.

4) In another smaller container, prepare the dressing by mixing the balsamic vinegar, olive oil and honey. Season with salt and pepper to taste. Beat or shake the mixture well until combined.

5) Drizzle the dressing over the salad and toss gently to make sure all the ingredients are coated.

6) Serve the spinach, strawberry, and walnut salad immediately.

Preparation time: Approximately 15 minutes.

Servings: 4 people

Chicken curry with vegetables and coconut milk

Ingredients:

- 500 grams of chicken breast cut into pieces

- 1 tablespoon olive oil

- 1 chopped onion

- 2 cloves of garlic, minced

- 1 tablespoon grated ginger

- 1 tablespoon curry powder

- 1 teaspoon turmeric powder

- 1 red pepper cut into strips

- 1 carrot cut into slices

- 200 grams of sliced mushrooms

- 1 can (400 ml) of coconut milk

- Salt and pepper to taste

- Chopped fresh cilantro to decorate (optional)

Instructions:

1) Heat the olive oil in a large skillet over medium-high heat. Add the onion and cook until translucent.

2) Add the garlic and grated ginger to the pan and cook for another minute.

3) Add the chicken cut into pieces and cook until golden brown on all sides.

4) Add the curry powder and turmeric and stir well so that the chicken is coated with the spices.

5) Add the red pepper, carrot, and mushrooms to the pan, and cook for about 5 minutes, until the vegetables are slightly tender.

6) Pour the coconut milk into the pan and mix well. Reduce the heat to medium-low and cook for another 10-15 minutes, until the chicken is cooked through, and the vegetables are tender.

7) Taste the seasoning and add salt and pepper to taste.

8) Serve the chicken curry with vegetables and coconut milk over brown rice or quinoa. If desired, garnish with fresh chopped cilantro.

Preparation time: Approximately 30 minutes.

Servings: 4 people

Beef stew with mushrooms and onion

Ingredients:

- 500 grams of beef in pieces

- 1 tablespoon olive oil

- 1 large onion cut into julienne strips

- 2 cloves of garlic, minced

- 200 grams of sliced mushrooms

- 1 large carrot cut into slices

- 2 cups low sodium beef broth

- 1 teaspoon dried rosemary

- 1 teaspoon dried thyme

- Salt and pepper to taste

• Chopped fresh parsley to decorate (optional)

Instructions:

1) In a large pot, heat the olive oil over medium-high heat. Add the beef and cook until golden brown on all sides.

2) Add the chopped onion and garlic to the pot and cook until the onion is translucent and fragrant.

3) Add the mushrooms and carrot slices to the pot and cook for a few minutes until the vegetables are slightly tender.

4) Pour the meat broth into the pot and add the rosemary and dried thyme. Stir well and bring the mixture to a boil.

5) Reduce the heat to medium-low, cover the pot, and let the stew cook for about 1 hour, or until the meat is tender and falls apart easily with a fork.

6) Taste the seasoning and add salt and pepper to taste.

7) Serve the beef stew with mushrooms and onion hot. If desired, garnish with fresh chopped parsley.

Preparation time: Approximately 1 hour and 15 minutes.

Servings: 4 people

Beet and feta salad

Ingredients:

• 4 medium beets cooked and cut into cubes

• 100 grams of crumbled feta cheese

• 1 cup mixed greens (lettuce, spinach, arugula, etc.)

• 1/4 cup chopped walnuts

• 2 tablespoons balsamic vinegar

• 2 tablespoons of olive oil

• Salt and pepper to taste

Instructions:

1) In a large bowl, combine the diced beets, crumbled feta cheese, and mixed greens.

2) Sprinkle the chopped walnuts over the salad.

3) In a separate container, mix the balsamic vinegar, olive oil, salt, and pepper.

4) Pour the dressing over the salad and mix gently to combine all the ingredients.

5) Serve the beet and feta salad on individual plates and enjoy.

Preparation time: Approximately 15 minutes.

Servings: 4 people

Grilled salmon with tomato and avocado salad

Ingredients:

• 4 fresh salmon fillets

• 2 tablespoons of olive oil

• Salt and pepper to taste

• 4 medium tomatoes, sliced

• 2 ripe avocados, cut into cubes

• 1 small red onion, cut into thin slices

• Juice of 1 lemon

• Fresh basil leaves to decorate

Instructions:

1) Preheat the grill to medium-high heat.

2) Brush the salmon fillets with olive oil and season with salt and pepper to taste.

3) Place the salmon fillets on the preheated grill and cook for approximately 4-5 minutes on each side, or until cooked to your preference.

4) Meanwhile, in a separate bowl, combine the tomato slices, avocado cubes, and red onion slices.

5) Drizzle the lemon juice over the salad and toss gently to combine the ingredients.

6) Remove the salmon from the grill and serve it along with the tomato and avocado salad.

7) Decorate with fresh basil leaves.

Preparation time: Approximately 20 minutes.

Servings: 4 people

This recipe gives you healthy and delicious option rich in omega-3 fatty acids and antioxidants.

Tomato soup with basil and oregano

Ingredients:

- 1 kg of ripe tomatoes, cut into pieces

- 1 large onion, chopped

- 2 cloves of garlic, minced

- 2 tablespoons of olive oil

- 4 cups low sodium vegetable broth

- 1 teaspoon dried oregano

- 1/2 cup fresh basil, chopped

- Salt and pepper to taste

• Fresh basil leaves to decorate

Instructions:

1) In a large pot, heat the olive oil over medium heat. Add the onion and garlic and cook until tender and fragrant.

2) Add the cut tomatoes to the pot and season with salt and pepper to taste. Cook for a few minutes until the tomatoes begin to soften.

3) Pour the vegetable broth into the pot and add the dried oregano. Bring the mixture to a boil and then reduce the heat to medium-low. Cook covered for about 20 minutes, so the flavors blend and the tomatoes break down.

4) Remove the pot from the heat and add the chopped fresh basil. Mix well.

5) Using a handheld blender or in a conventional blender, process the soup until you obtain a smooth and homogeneous consistency.

6) Reheat the soup over medium heat before serving.

7) Serve the tomato soup with basil and oregano hot. Decorate with fresh basil leaves.

Preparation time: Approximately 30 minutes.

Servings: 4 people

Roasted chicken with coleslaw

Ingredients:

• 4 pieces of chicken (thighs, breasts, or a combination)

• 2 tablespoons of olive oil

• 1 teaspoon smoked paprika

• 1 teaspoon garlic powder

• 1 teaspoon salt

• 1/2 teaspoon black pepper

- 1/2 medium white cabbage, grated or cut into thin strips

- 1 large carrot, grated

- 1/4 cup chopped fresh cilantro

- 2 tablespoons of lemon juice

- 2 tablespoons of apple cider vinegar

- 1 tablespoon of honey or natural sweetener (optional)

- Salt and pepper to taste

Instructions:

1) Preheat the oven to 200°C.

2) In a small bowl, mix the olive oil, smoked paprika, garlic powder, salt, and pepper.

3) Spread the chicken with this spice mixture on all sides.

4) Place the chicken on a baking sheet and roast in the preheated oven for approximately 45-50 minutes, or until cooked and golden.

5) Meanwhile, in a large bowl, combine the shredded cabbage, shredded carrot, and fresh cilantro.

6) In another smaller bowl, mix the lemon juice, apple cider vinegar, honey, or sweetener (optional), salt and pepper. Pour this mixture over the coleslaw and mix well so that the flavors integrate.

7) Once the chicken is ready, remove it from the oven and let it rest for a few minutes before cutting it into portions.

8) Serve the roast chicken along with the coleslaw.

Preparation time: Approximately 1 hour.

Servings: 4 people

This recipe gives you a healthy and tasty option, with the roasted chicken packed with lean protein and the coleslaw rich in nutrients.

Fish tacos with coleslaw

Ingredients:

- 500 grams of white fish fillets (such as cod or tilapia)

- 2 tablespoons of olive oil

- 2 teaspoons smoked paprika

- 1 teaspoon ground cumin

- 1 teaspoon garlic powder

- 1 teaspoon salt

- 1/2 teaspoon black pepper

- 1/4 red cabbage, cut into thin strips

- 1 large carrot, grated

- 1/4 cup chopped fresh cilantro

- Juice of 1 lemon

- 8 corn tortillas or whole wheat tortillas

- Yogurt sauce (optional)

Instructions:

1) In a small bowl, mix the olive oil, smoked paprika, cumin, garlic powder, salt, and pepper.

2) Spread the fish fillets with this spice mixture on both sides.

3) Heat a large skillet over medium-high heat and place the fish fillets in the hot skillet. Cook for about 3-4 minutes per side, or until the fish is cooked through and flakes easily.

4) Meanwhile, in a large bowl, combine the shredded red cabbage, grated carrot, and fresh cilantro.

5) Squeeze the lemon juice over the cabbage salad and mix well so that the flavors are integrated.

6) Heat the tortillas in a hot pan or in the oven.

7) Once the fish is ready, break it into smaller pieces.

8) Fill each tortilla with the shredded fish pieces and the cabbage salad. If you wish, add yogurt sauce for an additional touch.

9) Serve the fish tacos with slaw and enjoy.

Preparation time: Approximately 30 minutes.

Servings: 4 people

Anti-inflammatory desserts: In this section you will find delicious dessert recipes designed not only to satisfy the palate, but also to calm inflammatory processes at their source. All preparations have been made based on proven anti-inflammatory foods.

Here you can enjoy fresh antioxidant fruit smoothies, puddings and custards that soothe the digestive system and help your overall well-being. Desserts do not have to be the enemy of healthy eating. So, we invite you to explore these delicious desserts to pamper your body while pleasing your palate.

Yogurt ice cream with fresh fruits

Ingredients:

- 2 cups of natural yogurt

- 2 cups of fresh fruits cut into cubes (such as strawberries, pineapple, mango, melon, etc.)

- 1 tablespoon of honey

- 1 teaspoon vanilla extract

- 1 teaspoon grated ginger

- 1 teaspoon cinnamon powder

Instructions:

1) In a large bowl, mix the yogurt, honey, vanilla extract, grated ginger, and cinnamon powder until well combined.

2) Add the fresh fruits and stir until completely covered in the yogurt mixture.

3) Place the mixture in an ice cream mold and freeze for at least 3 hours or until firm.

4) Once the ice cream is completely frozen, remove it from the freezer and allow it to soften for a few minutes before serving. If desired, garnish with some additional fresh fruit before serving.

Preparation time: 10 minutes (plus 3 hours to freeze the ice cream).

Servings: 4 people

Oatmeal cookies with nuts and cinnamon.

Ingredients:

- 1 cup of oats

- 1/4 cup almond flour

- 1/4 cup honey

- 1/4 cup coconut oil

- 1/2 teaspoon cinnamon powder

- 1/4 cup of chopped nuts (such as almonds, walnuts, hazelnuts, etc.)

- 1/4 teaspoon salt

Instructions:

1) Preheat the oven to 180°C.

2) In a large bowl, mix the oats, almond flour, cinnamon, and salt.

3) Add the honey and coconut oil and mix well until you obtain a uniform dough.

4) Add the chopped nuts to the dough and mix again.

5) Form small balls with the dough and flatten them with the palm of your hand to give them a cookie shape.

6) Place the cookies on a baking sheet covered with parchment paper and bake for about 12-15 minutes or until golden brown.

7) Remove the cookies from the oven and let cool before serving.

Preparation time: 15 minutes.

Cooking time: 12-15 minutes.

Servings: 4 people

Apple pie with cinnamon

Ingredients:

- 1 pie dough (you can use a purchased pie dough or make it at home)

- 3 apples, peeled, seeded, and cut into thin slices

- 2 tablespoons of honey

- 1 teaspoon cinnamon powder

- 1 teaspoon grated ginger

- 1/4 cup chopped walnuts

- 1 tablespoon of almond flour

- 1 beaten egg

Instructions:

1) Preheat the oven to 180°C.

2) Place the pie dough in a pie pan and press gently to fit the pan tightly.

3) In a large bowl, mix the apples with the honey, cinnamon, and grated ginger.

4) Add the chopped walnuts and almond flour to the apple mixture and stir well.

5) Pour the apple mixture over the pie dough and distribute evenly.

6) Fold the edges of the pie dough inward to partially cover the edges of the apple mixture.

7) Paint the edges of the dough with the beaten egg.

8) Bake for about 40-45 minutes or until the dough is golden and crispy.

9) Remove from the oven and let cool before serving.

Preparation time: 20 minutes.

Cooking time: 40-45 minutes.

Servings: 4 people

Tropical fruit sorbet

Ingredients:

• 2 cups of frozen tropical fruits (such as mango, pineapple, papaya, etc.)

• 1 cup of fresh orange juice

• 1/4 cup honey

• 1 teaspoon grated ginger

• 1 teaspoon fresh lemon juice

Instructions:

1) Place the frozen tropical fruits in a blender or food processor.

2) Add the orange juice, honey, grated ginger and lemon juice to the blender or food processor.

3) Mix everything until you obtain a smooth and creamy mixture.

4) If the mixture is too thick, add a little more orange juice.

5) Serve immediately as a soft sorbet or freeze in an airtight container for 1-2 hours for a firmer sorbet.

6) Before serving, let the sorbet thaw slightly at room temperature.

Preparation time: 10 minutes.

Cooling time: 1-2 hours (optional).

Servings: 4 people

Black chocolate mousse

Ingredients:

• 200g of dark chocolate with a minimum of 70% cocoa

• 2 tablespoons of coconut oil

- 1/4 cup almond milk

- 1/4 cup honey

- 1 teaspoon vanilla

- 2 egg whites

- Pinch of salt

Instructions:

1) Melt the dark chocolate together with the coconut oil in a double boiler or in the microwave in 30 second intervals, stirring each time until completely melted.

2) Add the almond milk, honey and vanilla to the melted chocolate and mix well until combined.

3) Beat the egg whites with a pinch of salt until firm peaks form.

4) Add the beaten egg whites to the melted chocolate and mix gently until everything is combined.

5) Divide the mixture among four mousse molds and refrigerate for at least 2 hours or until firm.

Preparation time: 15 minutes.

Cooling time: 2 hours.

Servings: 4 people

Carrot and walnut cake

Ingredients:

- 2 cups of grated carrots

- 1 cup of almond flour

- 1/2 cup coconut flour

- 1/2 cup chopped walnuts

- 1/2 cup coconut oil

- 1/2 cup of honey

- 3 eggs

- 1 teaspoon baking soda

- 1 teaspoon cinnamon powder

- 1/2 teaspoon ginger powder

- 1/2 teaspoon nutmeg

- Pinch of salt

Instructions:

1) Preheat the oven to 180°C.

2) In a large bowl, mix the almond flour, coconut flour, baking soda, cinnamon, ginger, nutmeg and a pinch of salt.

3) In another bowl, beat the eggs and add the honey and melted coconut oil. Mix well.

4) Add the egg mixture to the dry ingredients and mix until everything is combined.

5) Add the grated carrots and chopped walnuts and mix well.

6) Pour the mixture into a previously greased cake pan.

7) Bake for 35-40 minutes or until the cake is golden brown and a toothpick inserted into the center comes out clean.

8) Let cool before cutting into portions.

Preparation time: 20 minutes.

Cooking time: 35-40 minutes.

Servings: 4 people

Greek yogurt with granola and fresh fruits

Ingredients:

• 2 cups of Greek yogurt

• 1 cup of granola

• 1 cup of fresh fruits (you can use whatever you prefer, such as strawberries, blueberries, kiwi, etc.)

• 1 tablespoon of honey (optional)

Instructions:

1) In a bowl, mix the Greek yogurt with the honey, if you want to sweeten it a little.

2) Into four serving bowls, divide Greek yogurt mixture evenly.

3) On top of the yogurt, add the granola in equal parts.

4) Next, add the fresh fruits cut into pieces on top of the granola, distributing them evenly among the four containers.

5) Serve cold.

Preparation time: 5 minutes.

Servings: 4 people

Roasted fruit with honey and cinnamon

Ingredients:

• 4 cups of fruit cut into pieces (you can use apples, pears, peaches, nectarines, bananas, or any fruit you prefer)

• 2 tablespoons of honey

• 1 teaspoon ground cinnamon

Instructions:

1) Preheat the oven to 180°C.

2) In a large bowl, mix the fruit with the honey and cinnamon, making sure all the fruit pieces are well coated.

3) Spread the fruit on a baking sheet.

4) Bake for 20-25 minutes or until the fruit is soft and golden.

5) Serve hot.

Preparation time: 10 minutes

Cooking time: 20-25 minutes

Servings: 4 people

Chia pudding with fresh fruits

Ingredients:

• 1/2 cup chia seeds

• 2 cups of milk (you can use almond milk or coconut milk for a vegan option)

• 2 tablespoons of honey

• 1 teaspoon vanilla extract

• 1 cup of fresh fruits (you can use whatever you prefer, such as strawberries, blueberries, kiwi, etc.)

• 1/4 cup chopped walnuts (optional)

Instructions:

1) In a large bowl, mix chia seeds, milk, honey, and vanilla extract. Mix well and let sit for at least 30 minutes or until the mixture thickens.

2) Once the mixture is thick, divide the chia pudding among four serving bowls.

3) On top of the chia pudding, add the fresh fruits cut into pieces.

4) If you want, add the chopped nuts on top of the fruits.

5) Serve cold.

Preparation time: 5 minutes

Standing time: 30 minutes

Servings: 4 people

Banana smoothie with cocoa powder

Ingredients:

- 2 ripe bananas

- 2 cups of unsweetened almond milk

- 2 tablespoons unsweetened cocoa powder

- 1 teaspoon ground cinnamon

- 1 teaspoon grated ginger

- 1 teaspoon honey (optional)

Instructions:

1) Peel the bananas and cut them into small pieces.

2) Place the bananas in a blender along with the almond milk, cocoa powder, ground cinnamon and grated ginger.

3) Mix all the ingredients until smooth and creamy.

4) If you want the smoothie to be a little sweeter, add a teaspoon of honey and mix again.

5) Pour the smoothie into glasses and serve immediately.

Preparation time: 10 minutes.

Servings: 4 people

Cheesecake with berries

Ingredients:

- 200 g low-fat cream cheese

- 2 eggs

- 1 tablespoon of honey

- 1 tablespoon fresh lemon juice

- 1 Teaspoon vanilla extract

- 100 g of fresh or frozen mixed berries

- 1 cup chopped walnuts

- 2 tablespoons of coconut oil

- 1 cup pitted dates

Instructions:

1) Preheat the oven to 180°C.

2) In a food processor, mix the walnuts, dates, and coconut oil until forming a uniform dough. Line a cake pans with the dough.

3) In a large bowl, beat the cream cheese, eggs, honey, lemon juice and vanilla essence until smooth.

4) Pour the cream cheese mixture into the base of the cake and add the berries on top.

5) Bake the cake for 20-25 minutes or until golden and firm to the touch.

6) Let cool and serve.

Preparation time: Approximately 30 minutes plus baking time in the oven.

Servings: 4 people

Vanilla flan with dried fruits

Ingredients:

- 2 cups of unsweetened almond milk

- 1/4 cup honey

- 3 eggs

- 1 teaspoon vanilla extract

- 1/4 cup chopped walnuts

- 1/4 cup chopped almonds

- 1/4 cup chopped hazelnuts

- 1 tablespoon of coconut oil

Instructions:

1) Preheat the oven to 180°C.

2) In a bowl, beat the eggs and honey until smooth.

3) Add the almond milk and vanilla extract and mix well.

4) In a frying pan, toast the walnuts, almonds, and hazelnuts with coconut oil until golden. Let cool and reserve.

5) Pour the egg mixture into a previously greased flan mold and sprinkle the toasted nuts on top.

6) Bake for 35-40 minutes or until the flan is firm to the touch.

7) Let cool and refrigerate for at least 2 hours before serving.

Preparation time: Approximately 20 minutes plus baking time in the oven (35-40 minutes) and refrigeration (minimum 2 hours)

Servings: 4 people

Black bean and dark chocolate brownie

Ingredients:

- 1 can of black beans, drained and rinsed
- 1/4 cup coconut oil
- 2 eggs
- 1/2 cup oat flour
- 1/2 cup unsweetened cocoa powder
- 1/2 cup of honey
- 1 teaspoon vanilla extract
- 1/2 teaspoon baking powder
- 1/4 teaspoon salt
- 1/2 cup chopped dark chocolate

Instructions:

1) Preheat the oven to 180°C.

2) In a food processor, blend the black beans and coconut oil until they form a smooth paste.

3) Add the eggs and mix until there is a homogeneous mixture.

4) Add the oat flour, cocoa powder, honey, vanilla extract, baking powder and salt. Mix well until you have a smooth dough.

5) Add the chopped dark chocolate to the mixture.

6) Pour the mixture into a previously greased baking pan.

7) Bake for 25-30 minutes or until the brownie is firm to the touch.

8) Let cool before cutting into portions.

Preparation time: approximately 15 minutes plus baking time in the oven (25-30 minutes)

Portions. 4 people

Fruit salad with yogurt and honey

Ingredients:

• 2 cups of assorted fruits (for example: strawberries, kiwis, mangoes, pineapples, bananas, etc.), cut into small pieces

• 1 cup unsweetened Greek yogurt

• 2 tablespoons of honey

• 1 teaspoon ground cinnamon

• 1/4 cup chopped walnuts (optional)

Instructions:

1) In a large bowl, mix the chopped fruits.

2) In another bowl, mix the Greek yogurt, honey, and cinnamon until smooth.

3) Pour the yogurt mixture over the fruits and mix gently until the fruits are well coated.

4) Sprinkle the chopped walnuts on top (optional).

5) Serve immediately or store in the refrigerator until serving time.

Preparation time: approximately 10 minutes.

Servings: 4 people

Tofu dessert with fruits and honey

Ingredients:

• 1 block of firm tofu (350g), drained and cut into small cubes

• 2 tablespoons of honey

• 1 teaspoon vanilla extract

• 1/4 cup unsweetened almond milk

• 2 cups of assorted fruits (for example: strawberries, blueberries, kiwis, mango, etc.), cut into small pieces

• 1 tablespoon chia seeds (optional)

Instructions:

1) In a food processor, blend the tofu, honey, vanilla extract, and almond milk until smooth.

2) Divide the tofu mixture among 4 dessert glasses.

3) Cover each glass with a layer of chopped fruits.

4) Repeat layers until all fruits and tofu have been used.

5) Sprinkle chia seeds on top (optional).

6) Serve immediately or store in the refrigerator until serving time.

Preparation time: approximately 15 minutes.

Servings: 4 people

Mango mousse with yogurt

Ingredients:

• 2 ripe mangoes, peeled and cut into pieces

• 1 cup unsweetened Greek yogurt

• 2 tablespoons of honey

• 1 teaspoon vanilla extract

• 1 tablespoon fresh lemon juice

• 1 sachet of unflavored gelatin

- 1/4 cup hot water

Instructions:

1) In a food processor or blender, blend the mango pieces until you obtain a smooth puree.

2) In a large bowl, mix the mango puree, Greek yogurt, honey, vanilla extract and lemon juice.

3) In another small bowl, mix the unflavored gelatin and hot water until completely dissolved.

4) Add the dissolved gelatin to the mango and yogurt mixture and mix well.

5) Divide the mousse mixture among 4 dessert glasses.

6) Refrigerate for at least 2 hours so the mousse sets.

7) Decorate with fresh fruits and serve cold.

Preparation time: approximately 20 minutes, plus 2 hours of refrigeration.

Servings: 4 people

Almond and dark chocolate truffles

Ingredients:

- 1/2 cup raw almonds
- 1/4 cup coconut flakes
- 1/4 cup chopped dark chocolate
- 1 tablespoon of coconut oil
- 1 tablespoon of honey
- 1/4 teaspoon ground cinnamon
- A pinch of sea salt

Instructions:

1) In a food processor, mix the almonds and coconut flakes until you obtain a fine mixture.

2) Add the chopped dark chocolate, coconut oil, honey, cinnamon, and sea salt, and mix well.

3) Form small balls with the mixture and place them on a plate lined with wax paper.

4) Freeze the truffles for at least 30 minutes before serving.

5) Garnish with additional almonds or coconut flakes before serving, if desired.

Preparation time: approximately 20 minutes, plus 30 minutes freezing.

Servings: 4 people

Strawberry and kiwi smoothie

Ingredients:

• 2 cups fresh strawberries, washed and cut into quarters

• 2 kiwis peeled and cut into pieces

• 1 ripe banana, peeled and cut into slices

• 1 cup unsweetened Greek yogurt

• 1/2 cup unsweetened almond milk

• 1 tablespoon of honey

• 1 teaspoon vanilla extract

• 1 cup of ice

Instructions:

1) In a blender, blend the strawberries, kiwis, banana, Greek yogurt, almond milk, honey, vanilla extract, and ice until you obtain a smooth and creamy shake.

2) If the smoothie is too thick, add a little more almond milk until it has the desired consistency.

3) Divide the smoothie into 4 glasses to serve.

4) Decorate with fresh fruits before serving, if desired.

Preparation time: approximately 10 minutes.

Servings: 4 people

Pumpkin and walnut cake

Ingredients:

- 1 cup pumpkin puree

- 1/2 cup melted coconut oil

- 1/2 cup of honey

- 2 eggs

- 1 teaspoon vanilla extract

- 1 1/2 cups oat flour

- 1 teaspoon baking soda

- 1/2 teaspoon baking powder

- 1 teaspoon ground cinnamon

- 1/4 teaspoon ground nutmeg

- 1/4 teaspoon sea salt

- 1/2 cup chopped walnuts

Instructions:

1) Preheat the oven to 180°C. Grease a 20cm cake tin.

2) In a large bowl, mix the pumpkin puree, melted coconut oil, honey, eggs and vanilla extract.

3) In another bowl, mix the oat flour, baking soda, baking powder, ground cinnamon, ground nutmeg and sea salt.

4) Gradually add the flour mixture to the pumpkin mixture, stirring until well combined.

5) Add the chopped walnuts and mix well.

6) Pour the mixture into the prepared pan and bake for about 40-45 minutes, or until a toothpick inserted into the center of the cake comes out clean.

7) Let cool in the mold for a few minutes before removing and cooling completely on a wire rack.

Preparation time: approximately 20 minutes, plus 40-45 minutes of baking.

Servings: 4 people

<u>Gingerbread and cinnamon cookies</u>

Ingredients:

- 1 cup of almond flour

- 1/2 cup coconut flour

- 1/4 cup honey

- 1 egg

- 2 teaspoons of ground ginger

- 2 teaspoons of ground cinnamon

- 1/2 teaspoon baking soda

- 1/4 teaspoon sea salt

- 1/4 cup melted coconut oil

Instructions:

1) Preheat the oven to 180°C. Line a baking sheet with parchment paper.

2) In a large bowl, mix the almond flour, coconut flour, honey, egg, ground ginger, ground cinnamon, baking soda and sea salt.

3) Add the melted coconut oil and mix well until you obtain a soft dough.

4) Form the dough into small balls, place them on the prepared baking sheet and flatten them slightly with a spatula or fork.

5) Bake for about 10-12 minutes or until golden.

6) Let cool completely on the tray before serving.

Preparation time: approximately 20 minutes, plus 10-12 minutes of baking.

Servings: 4 people

Banana ice cream with almonds

Ingredients:

• 4 ripe bananas

• 1/2 cup almond milk

• 1 teaspoon vanilla extract

• 1/4 cup chopped almonds

• 1 tablespoon of honey (optional)

Instructions:

1) Peel the bananas and cut them into small pieces. Freeze the banana pieces for at least 2 hours.

2) Once the bananas are frozen, place them in a food processor or blender along with the almond milk and vanilla extract. Mix well until the mixture has a smooth and creamy consistency.

3) Add the chopped almonds to the mixture and mix gently.

4) If you want a sweeter flavor, add honey to the mixture and mix well.

5) Transfer the mixture to a freezer-safe container and freeze for at least 2 hours or until the ice cream is firm.

6) To serve, remove the ice cream from the freezer and let it sit at room temperature for a few minutes to soften a little before serving.

Preparation time: approximately 10 minutes, plus 2 hours of freezing.

Servings: 4 people

Cheesecake and blueberries

Ingredients:

- 1 cup fresh or frozen blueberries

- 1 cup low-fat cream cheese

- 1/2 cup low-fat Greek yogurt

- 1/4 cup honey

- 2 eggs

- 1 teaspoon vanilla extract

- 1/2 cup oat flour

- 1/4 cup chopped almonds

- 1 teaspoon ground cinnamon

- 1/4 teaspoon salt

Instructions:

1) Preheat the oven to 180°C and grease a 20 cm diameter cake pan.

2) Place the cranberries in a small skillet over medium-high heat and cook until they soften and small bubbles form. Remove from heat and let cool.

3) In a large bowl, beat cream cheese, Greek yogurt, and honey until smooth.

4) Add the eggs and vanilla extract to the mixture and beat until well incorporated.

5) In another bowl, mix the oat flour, chopped almonds, ground cinnamon and salt. Add the flour mixture to the cream cheese mixture and beat until all ingredients are incorporated.

6) Pour the cheese mixture into the prepared pan and spread the blueberries on top.

7) Bake for 30-35 minutes, or until the cake is golden brown and firm in the center.

8) Let the cake cool for 10-15 minutes before serving.

Preparation time: approximately 15 minutes, plus 30-35 minutes of baking.

Servings: 4 people

Cinnamon rice pudding

Ingredients:

- 1 cup of brown rice

- 2 cups of water

- 1 cup of almond milk

- 2 teaspoons of ground cinnamon

- 2 tablespoons of honey

- 1 teaspoon vanilla extract

Preparation:

1) Rinse the rice in a colander and put it in a medium saucepan with water. Bring to a boil, then reduce the heat and simmer for about 40 minutes, or until tender and the water has been absorbed.

2) Add the almond milk, cinnamon, honey, and vanilla extract to the cooked rice and mix well.

3) Cook over medium heat, stirring constantly, for about 5 minutes or until the mixture thickens.

4) Remove from heat and let cool for a few minutes before serving.

5) Serve in individual bowls and sprinkle a little ground cinnamon on top if you wish.

Preparation time: Approximately 50 minutes.

Servings: 4 people

Coconut flan with fresh fruits

Ingredients:

- 1 can of coconut milk (400ml)

- 1 cup of skimmed milk

- 1/2 cup coconut sugar

- 3 eggs

- 1/2 cup of grated coconut meat

- 1 teaspoon vanilla extract

- Fresh fruits to taste (strawberries, mango, kiwi, etc.)

Instructions:

1) Preheat the oven to 180°C.

2) In a medium saucepan, mix the coconut milk, skimmed milk, and coconut sugar. Heat over medium heat until the sugar is completely dissolved.

3) In a large bowl, beat the eggs with the grated coconut meat and vanilla extract.

4) Add the hot milk mixture to the egg mixture little by little, whisking constantly.

5) Strain the mixture to eliminate lumps and pour into a flan mold.

6) Fill a baking dish with hot water and place the flan mold inside it.

7) Bake for 45-50 minutes, or until the flan is set, but still slightly jiggly.

8) Remove the mold from the water and let it cool to room temperature.

9) Refrigerate for at least 2 hours before serving.

10) Serve the coconut flan with the fresh fruits cut into cubes or slices.

Preparation time: 15 minutes

Cooking time: 50 minutes

Cooling time: 2 hours

Servings: 4 people

Red fruit smoothie with yogurt

Ingredients:

• 2 cups of frozen red fruits (strawberries, raspberries, blackberries)

• 1 cup of non-fat natural yogurt

• 1 cup unsweetened almond milk

• 1 teaspoon grated ginger

• 1 teaspoon honey (optional)

• 4 ice cubes

Instructions:

1) In a blender, mix the frozen berries, yogurt, almond milk, grated ginger, and honey (if using).

2) Add the ice cubes to the blender and blend on high speed for 1-2 minutes or until the mixture is smooth and homogeneous.

3) Serve the smoothie immediately in 4 glasses. You can decorate with a strawberry or a mint leaf if you wish.

Prep Time: Prep time for this recipe is approximately 5-10 minutes, depending on the speed of your blender and whether you have the ingredients already measured and ready to use.

Servings: 4 people

Pear and almond cake

Ingredients:

- 1 ripe pear, peeled and thinly sliced

- 1 cup of ground almonds

- 1/2 cup oat flour

- 1/4 cup melted coconut oil

- 1/4 cup of honey

- 2 large eggs

- 1 teaspoon vanilla extract

- 1/2 teaspoon ground cinnamon

- 1/4 teaspoon ground nutmeg

- A pinch of salt

Instructions:

1) Preheat the oven to 180°C. Grease a 20cm diameter cake pan with coconut oil and sprinkle with oat flour.

2) In a large bowl, mix the ground almonds, oat flour, ground cinnamon, ground nutmeg and a pinch of salt.

3) In another bowl, beat the eggs with the melted coconut oil, honey, and vanilla extract until you obtain a smooth and homogeneous mixture.

4) Add the liquid ingredients to the dry ingredients and mix well until a uniform dough is formed.

5) Pour the batter into the prepared pan and spread it evenly on the bottom.

6) Place the pear slices on top of the dough, pressing them down slightly.

7) Bake the cake for 30-35 minutes or until golden brown and firm to the touch.

8) Let the cake cool before serving.

Prep Time: Prep time for this recipe is approximately 15-20 minutes, and cooking time is 30-35 minutes. So, in total, this recipe should take about 45-55 minutes to prepare and cook.

Servings: 4 people

Beetroot and dark chocolate brownie

Ingredients:

• 1 large beet, peeled and finely grated

• 1 cup of almond flour

• 1/2 cup oat flour

• 1/4 cup unsweetened cocoa powder

• 1/4 cup of honey

• 1/4 cup melted coconut oil

• 2 large eggs

• 1 teaspoon vanilla extract

• 1/2 teaspoon baking soda

• 1/4 teaspoon salt

• 1/2 cup unsweetened dark chocolate chips

Instructions:

1) Preheat the oven to 180°C. Grease a 20cm diameter brownie pan with coconut oil and sprinkle with oat flour.

2) In a large bowl, mix the almond flour, oat flour, cocoa powder, baking soda and pinch of salt.

3) In another bowl, beat the eggs with the melted coconut oil, honey, and vanilla extract until you obtain a smooth and homogeneous mixture.

4) Add the liquid ingredients to the dry ingredients and mix well until a uniform dough is formed.

5) Add the grated beet to the dough and mix well to incorporate it.

6) Add the dark chocolate chips and mix again.

7) Pour the batter into the prepared pan and spread it evenly on the bottom.

8) Bake the brownie for 25-30 minutes or until golden brown and firm to the touch.

9) Let the brownie cool before cutting it into portions.

Prep Time: Prep time for this recipe is approximately 20-25 minutes, and cooking time is 25-30 minutes. So, in total, this recipe should take about 45-55 minutes to prepare and cook.

Servings: 4 people

Fruit salad with yogurt and honey

Ingredients:

• 2 cups of chopped fresh fruits (can be strawberries, blueberries, kiwi, mango, pineapple, etc.)

• 1/2 cup of low-fat natural yogurt

- 2 tablespoons of honey

- 1 teaspoon lemon juice

- 1/4 cup slivered and toasted almonds

Instructions:

1) Wash and cut the fruits into small pieces and place them in a large bowl.

2) In a separate bowl, mix the yogurt, honey, and lemon juice until well combined.

3) Pour the yogurt mixture over the fruits and mix gently until all the fruits are covered with the yogurt.

4) Sprinkle the toasted almonds over the fruit salad.

5) Serve the fruit salad cold and enjoy.

Prep Time: Prep time for this recipe is approximately 10-15 minutes, and no cooking is required.

Servings: 4 people

Chia custard with fresh fruits

Ingredients:

- 1/4 cup chia seeds

- 1 1/2 cups unsweetened almond milk

- 2 tablespoons of honey

- 1 teaspoon vanilla extract

- Chopped fresh fruits (can be strawberries, kiwi, mango, etc.)

- 2 tablespoons of chopped walnuts (optional)

Instructions:

1) In a bowl, mix the chia seeds, almond milk, honey, and vanilla extract until well combined.

2) Cover the bowl with plastic wrap and refrigerate the mixture for at least 4 hours or overnight, until the mixture has thickened, and the chia seeds have hydrated.

3) Once the mixture has thickened, stir it well to make sure there are no lumps.

4) Serve the custard in bowls or glasses and add the chopped fresh fruits and chopped nuts on top.

5) Serve cold and enjoy.

Prep Time: Prep time for this recipe is about 5-10 minutes, but you should refrigerate the chia mixture for at least 4 hours before serving. So, in total, this recipe should take about 4-5 hours to prepare and be ready to serve.

Servings: 4 people

Pineapple mousse with yogurt

Ingredients:

- 1 cup chopped pineapple

- 1/2 cup low-fat Greek yogurt

- 2 tablespoons of honey

- 1 teaspoon lemon juice

- 1 teaspoon unflavored gelatin

- 1/4 cup hot water

- 1/4 cup whipped cream (optional)

Instructions:

1) In a blender, blend the pineapple, yogurt, honey, and lemon juice until the mixture is smooth.

2) In a small bowl, mix unflavored gelatin with hot water until gelatin is completely dissolved.

3) Add the dissolved gelatin to the pineapple mixture in the blender and mix well.

4) Pour the pineapple mousse mixture into bowls or glasses and refrigerate for at least 1 hour or until the mousse is firm.

5) If desired, add a dollop of whipped cream on top of each serving before serving.

Prep Time: Prep time for this recipe is about 10-15 minutes, but you should refrigerate the mousse for at least 1 hour before serving. So, in total, this recipe should take about 1 hour and 15 minutes to prepare and be ready to serve.

Servings: 4 people

Strawberry and pineapple smoothie with ginger

Ingredients:

• 2 cups fresh strawberries, cut into pieces

• 1 cup fresh pineapple, cut into pieces

• 1 teaspoon grated fresh ginger

• 1 cup unsweetened Greek yogurt

• 1 tablespoon of honey (optional, to sweeten)

Instructions:

1) In a blender, add the strawberries, pineapple, and grated ginger.

2) Mix the ingredients at high speed until you obtain a smooth and homogeneous mixture.

3) Add the Greek yogurt to the blender and blend again until all the ingredients are well combined.

4) If you want to sweeten the smoothie, add the honey, and mix again.

5) Once you achieve the desired consistency, pour the smoothie into glasses or serving containers.

Preparation time: Approximately 10 minutes.

Servings: 4 people.

Oat truffles and cocoa powder

Ingredients:

- 1 cup of rolled oats

- 1/2 cup almond butter

- 1/4 cup honey or agave syrup

- 2 tablespoons unsweetened cocoa powder

- 1 teaspoon vanilla extract

- 1/4 cup grated coconut (optional, to decorate)

Instructions:

1) In a food processor, pulse the oats until you obtain a fine texture.

2) Add the almond butter, honey or agave syrup, cocoa powder, and vanilla extract to the food processor.

3) Mix all the ingredients until you obtain a homogeneous and sticky dough.

4) Form small balls with the dough and place them on a plate or tray lined with wax paper.

5) If desired, roll the truffles in shredded coconut to decorate.

6) Refrigerate the truffles for at least 30 minutes before serving.

Preparation time: Approximately 20 minutes, plus refrigeration time of at least 30 minutes.

Servings: 4 people

Mango and banana smoothie

Ingredients:

• 2 ripe mangoes, peeled and pitted

• 2 ripe bananas

• 1 cup unsweetened coconut yogurt

• 1 cup unsweetened almond milk

• 1 teaspoon honey (optional, to sweeten)

• Ice cubes (optional)

Instructions:

1) Cut the mangoes and bananas into pieces.

2) In a blender, add the mangoes, bananas, coconut yogurt and almond milk.

3) Mix the ingredients on high speed until you obtain a smooth and creamy consistency.

4) If you want to sweeten the smoothie, add the honey, and mix again.

5) If you prefer a colder texture, add a few ice cubes, and mix again until well crushed.

6) Pour the smoothie into serving glasses.

Preparation time: Approximately 5 minutes.

Servings: 4 people

Lemon and chia seeds cake

Ingredients:

- 1 1/2 cups whole wheat flour

- 1/2 cup almond flour

- 1/4 cup chia seeds

- 2 teaspoons baking powder

- 1/2 teaspoon baking soda

- 1/4 teaspoon salt

- 1/2 cup honey or agave syrup

- 1/4 cup melted coconut oil

- 1/2 cup unsweetened almond milk

- Juice and zest of 2 lemons

- 2 eggs

- 1 teaspoon vanilla extract

Instructions:

1) Preheat the oven to 180°C (350°F) and grease a cake tin.

2) In a large bowl, whisk together whole wheat flour, almond flour, chia seeds, baking powder, baking soda, and salt.

3) In another bowl, combine honey or agave syrup, melted coconut oil, almond milk, lemon juice and zest, eggs, and vanilla extract. Mix all the liquid ingredients well.

4) Pour the liquid mixture into the bowl of dry ingredients and stir until a homogeneous dough forms.

5) Pour the batter into the prepared pan and smooth it out with a spatula.

6) Bake the cake for approximately 30-35 minutes, or until golden brown and a toothpick inserted into the center comes out clean.

7) Once baked, remove the cake from the oven and let it cool in the pan for a few minutes. Then transfer to a wire rack to cool completely.

Preparation time: Approximately 15 minutes.

Cooking time: Approximately 30-35 minutes.

Servings: 4 people

Coconut and nut cookies

Ingredients:

- 1 1/2 cups unsweetened shredded coconut

- 1/2 cup of chopped nuts (almonds, walnuts, hazelnuts, etc.)

- 1/4 cup chia seeds

- 2 tablespoons honey or agave syrup

- 2 tablespoons of melted coconut oil

- 1 teaspoon vanilla extract

- 1 egg

Instructions:

1) Preheat the oven to 180°C (350°F) and line a baking sheet with wax paper.

2) In a bowl, mix the grated coconut, chopped nuts and chia seeds.

3) In another bowl, whisk together the honey or agave syrup, melted coconut oil, vanilla extract, and egg. Beat all liquid ingredients until well combined.

4) Pour the liquid mixture into the bowl of dry ingredients and stir until all ingredients are completely incorporated.

5) Take portions of dough and form round cookies. Place them on the baking sheet, leaving enough space between them.

6) Lightly press each cookie with the back of a spoon to flatten it.

7) Bake the cookies for approximately 12-15 minutes, or until lightly golden around the edges.

8) Once baked, remove the cookies from the oven and let them cool completely on the tray before handling them.

Preparation time: 15 minutes.

Cooking time: Approximately 12-15 minutes.

Servings: 4 people.

Forest fruit ice cream

Ingredients:

- 2 cups of frozen berries (blueberries, raspberries, blackberries, etc.)
- 1 frozen ripe banana
- 1/2 cup unsweetened coconut milk
- 2 tablespoons of honey or agave syrup (optional, to sweeten)

Instructions:

1) Place the frozen berries, frozen banana, and coconut milk in a blender or food processor.

2) Mix the ingredients at high speed until you obtain a smooth and creamy mixture.

3) If you want to sweeten the ice cream, add the honey or agave syrup, and mix again.

4) Taste the mixture and adjust the sweetness level according to your preference.

5) Once you achieve the desired consistency, transfer the ice cream to a freezer-safe container.

6) Cover the container and place it in the freezer for at least 3-4 hours, or until the ice cream is firm.

7) Take the ice cream out of the freezer a few minutes before serving so that it softens slightly.

8) Serve the berry ice cream in bowls or cones and enjoy.

Preparation time: Approximately 10 minutes.

Freezing time: Approximately 3-4 hours.

Servings: 4 people.

Apple and cinnamon cake without sugar

Ingredients:

For the mass:

- 1 1/2 cups whole wheat flour

- 1/2 cup almond flour

- 1/4 cup melted coconut oil

- 1/4 cup cold water

- 1 teaspoon vanilla extract

For the filling:

- 4 large apples, peeled, cored, and cut into thin slices

- 2 teaspoons of cinnamon powder

- 1 tablespoon lemon juice

- Natural sweetener to taste (stevia, erythritol, etc.)

Instructions:

1) Preheat the oven to 180°C (350°F) and grease a cake tin.

2) In a large bowl, mix together whole wheat flour and almond flour.

3) Add the melted coconut oil, cold water, and vanilla extract to the bowl of dry ingredients. Mix until a dough forms.

4) Lightly flour a work surface and roll out the dough with a rolling pin until it is large enough to cover the tart pan.

5) Place the dough in the mold and press gently to cover it completely.

6) In a separate bowl, mix the apple slices, cinnamon powder, lemon juice and natural sweetener to taste. Make sure the apples are well coated with the cinnamon.

7) Distribute the apple slices in the mold over the dough, creating an even layer.

8) Bake the pie for approximately 35-40 minutes, or until the crust is golden brown and the apples are tender.

9) Once baked, remove the cake from the oven and let it cool before serving.

Preparation time: 20 minutes.

Cooking time: Approximately 35-40 minutes.

Servings: 4 people.

Chia pudding with coconut milk

Ingredients:

- 1/2 cup chia seeds

- 2 cups of unsweetened coconut milk

- 2 tablespoons of honey or agave syrup (optional, to sweeten)

- 1 teaspoon vanilla extract

- Fresh fruits to decorate (strawberries, blueberries, kiwi, etc.)

- Chopped nuts to decorate (almonds, walnuts, etc.)

Instructions:

1) In a large bowl, combine the chia seeds, coconut milk, honey, or agave syrup (if desired), and vanilla extract. Mix all ingredients well.

2) Stir the mixture for a few minutes to make sure the chia seeds are evenly distributed and no clumps form.

3) Cover the bowl and refrigerate the pudding for at least 2 hours, or until it has thickened and acquired a gelatinous texture.

4) Remove the chia pudding from the refrigerator and stir again before serving.

5) Divide the pudding into individual bowls or cups.

6) Decorate each serving with fresh fruit and chopped nuts.

7) Serve the chia pudding with coconut milk cold and enjoy.

Preparation time: Approximately 5 minutes.

Standing time: Approximately 2 hours.

Servings: 4 people.

Dark chocolate flan with walnuts

Ingredients:

• 3 cups of unsweetened almond milk

• 200 g dark chocolate (minimum 70% cocoa), chopped

• 1/2 cup chopped walnuts

• 1/2 cup of natural sweetener (stevia, erythritol, etc.)

• 4 eggs

• 1 teaspoon vanilla extract

Instructions:

1) Preheat the oven to 180°C (350°F).

2) In a saucepan, heat the almond milk over medium heat until hot but not boiling.

3) Remove the pot from the heat and add the chopped chocolate. Stir until the chocolate has completely melted and the mixture is smooth.

4) Add the chopped nuts and mix again.

5) In a separate bowl, beat the eggs, natural sweetener, and vanilla extract until smooth.

6) Slowly pour the egg mixture into the pot with the almond milk and chocolate, stirring constantly to prevent the eggs from cooking.

7) Once all the ingredients are well incorporated, pour the mixture into individual flan molds.

8) Place the molds on a baking tray and fill the tray with hot water until they reach half the height of the molds.

9) Bake for approximately 35-40 minutes, or until the flans are firm around the edges, but still have a slight jiggle in the center.

10) Remove the molds from the hot water and let the flans cool to room temperature.

11) Next, refrigerate the flans for at least 2 hours, or until they are completely cold and firm.

12) Once refrigerated, unmold the flans, and serve them cold.

Preparation time: 20 minutes.

Cooking time: Approximately 35-40 minutes.

Cooling time: Approximately 2 hours.

Servings: 4 people.

Banana and strawberry smoothie with almond milk

Ingredients:

- 2 ripe bananas

- 2 cups of fresh strawberries

- 2 cups of unsweetened almond milk

- 1 tablespoon honey or agave syrup (optional, to sweeten)

- Ice (optional, for a colder and thicker consistency)

Instructions:

1) Peel the bananas and cut them into slices.

2) Wash and cut the strawberries into pieces.

3) In a blender, add the bananas, strawberries, almond milk, and honey or agave syrup (if you want to sweeten the smoothie).

4) Optionally, add a few ice cubes to the blender if you want a colder, thicker consistency.

5) Blend all the ingredients at high speed until you obtain a smooth and homogeneous mixture.

6) Taste the smoothie and adjust the sweetness level by adding more honey or agave syrup, if necessary.

7) Once the smoothie is ready, serve it in glasses or glasses.

8) You can decorate the smoothie with a fresh strawberry on top if you wish.

9) Enjoy the Strawberry Banana Almond Milk Smoothie right away.

Preparation time: Approximately 5 minutes.

Portions. 4 people.

I sincerely hope that you have enjoyed cooking and trying all these preparations that we have lovingly selected for you. More than a simple recipe book, this book represents an invitation to take care of your health and well-being through one of the most pleasant acts: eating delicious and healthy food.

These 100 recipes that make up this work have the power to help reduce chronic inflammation, which translates into a better quality of life. Now they have delicious alternatives to easily implement an anti-inflammatory diet.

Remember to adjust the quantities of the ingredients according to the number of servings you need.